Managing Health and Safety
in the Dental Practice

Managing Health and Safety in the Dental Practice

A Practical Guide

Jane Bonehill, FRSPH, Tech IOSH, LiCIPD, AIfl

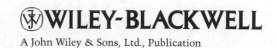

A John Wiley & Sons, Ltd., Publication

This edition first published 2010
© 2010 by Blackwell Publishing Ltd.

Blackwell Publishing was acquired by John Wiley & Sons in February 2007. Blackwell's publishing programme has been merged with Wiley's global Scientific, Technical, and Medical business to form Wiley-Blackwell.

Registered office
John Wiley & Sons Ltd, The Atrium, Southern Gate, Chichester, West Sussex, PO19 8SQ, United Kingdom

Editorial offices
9600 Garsington Road, Oxford, OX4 2DQ, United Kingdom
2121 State Avenue, Ames, Iowa 50014-8300, USA

For details of our global editorial offices, for customer services and for information about how to apply for permission to reuse the copyright material in this book please see our website at www.wiley.com/wiley-blackwell.

Library of Congress Cataloging-in-Publication Data

Bonehill, Jane A.
    Managing health and safety in the dental practice : a practical guide / Jane Bonehill.
        p. ; cm.
    Includes index.
    ISBN 978-1-4051-8592-9 (pbk. : alk. paper) 1. Dentistry – Safety measures. 2. Dental offices – Sanitation.
I. Title.
    [DNLM: 1. Practice Management, Dental – organization & administration. 2. Accidents,
Occupational – prevention & control. 3. Occupational Health Services – organization & administration.
4. Risk Assessment – methods. 5. Safety Management – methods. WU 77 B712m 2010]
    RK52.B66 2010
    617.60028′9 – dc22

                                                                                                    2010001840

A catalogue record for this book is available from the British Library.

Set in 10/12pt Sabon by Laserwords Private Limited, Chennai, India
Print and bound in Malaysia by Vivar Printing Sdn Bhd

1   2010

Contents

Dedication

Special thoughts go to Sister Carole. Her courage inspired me
to complete. This one is for you. xxx

Acknowledgements

I thank all the people who supported me during the months that this manual took to produce. Without their dedication and enthusiasm it would have been a seemingly impossible task.

In particular, I am forever grateful to my sister Tricia who painstakingly proofread all of the text in every chapter. Her expertise and feedback were essential for the content to be interpreted by the reader as it was intended.

My colleague and friend Clare Roberts must also have a mention; she once again stepped in when the going got tough, as did Susan Audrey who rallied round to do all the other tasks I should have been doing.

Last but not the least, my husband Keith really came up trumps, and reminded me of all the reasons why I married him.

Preface

It has long been recognised that the general consensus of opinion is that health and safety is not the most interesting of subjects. This is probably one of the reasons why in many organisations the approach to health and safety is somewhat reactive, that is, health and safety is only addressed when something happens. Some people call this 'fire fighting'. This approach not only has the potential to make the dental practice and the way we work unsafe but also leaves us wide open to the risk of legal action.

The author recognises the many 'hats' that practice managers wear and the difficulties this brings with it. Her experience shows that very few are specialists in the health and safety field. This manual has been developed in order to simplify the approach to the way you address health and safety in dental practice and to assist with the day-to-day management of this seemingly dull subject. The primary aim is to make health and safety as much of a priority as all your other business functions by integrating it into your overall management system. This will assist you in preventing accidents, addressing unacceptable working practices and maintaining professional standards in order to ensure, so far as is reasonable, the protection of employees and patients. Each chapter is structured to ensure that the subject contains sufficient details without overburdening you with technical information, is specific to the dental practice needs and is realistic, practical and achievable. Legal duties are stated in each chapter, together with an explanation of how these are applied. It should be recognised that legislation and codes of practice change from time to time; therefore, it is the responsibility of the practice to keep themselves abreast of these changes. It is also the author's intention to encourage a team approach by actively involving all members of the team in making health and safety work for you.

How to use this manual

The advantages of this manual are that you can pick it up and, using the index or chapter tabs, sort through to the essential 'need to' and 'should know' information from the 'might also want to know more about' information. It is not intended that you read this manual from cover to cover. However, it is advised that you read the next section 'Introduction – legal information'. This will provide an insight into how health and safety is regulated and the responsibilities placed on individuals.

The manual has been prepared in such a way that it guides you through the subject area. Each chapter is structured as follows:

- A **Graphic** depicting the topic for ease of reference
- A bulleted list outlining the **Scope** of the chapter
- A list of **Figures** placed at the beginning of the chapter
- An **Introduction** to the subject to set the scene and outline the purpose
- A list of key **Legislation** relating to the subject
- The subject **Content** broken down into sub-headings with reference to figures throughout the text
- A **Summary** to help reflection and to take on board the content
- **Action check list** to measure against your existing arrangements and working practices
- **Frequently asked questions** to assist with the practical application of the subject

- **Links to other chapters** for cross-referencing purposes

All members of the team, not just employers and managers, should use this manual.

Getting started

Familiarise yourself with the structure and format of this manual, and then study the index and identify the subjects, which in your practice, you feel, need addressing. At this stage, you will have just a 'gut feeling' and not an authoritative opinion. Then read through 'Introduction – legal information'. Following this you may want to hold a practice meeting with all members of your team and ask them to prepare for the meeting by identifying any issues or suggestions they have about health and safety. You may have to provide key indicators to help, which could relate to the following:

- A recent incident where a patient was difficult or aggressive
- The use of a particular piece of equipment
- Preparing a hazardous substance
- Posture when treating patients
- 'Good practice' that a colleague from another dental practice has shared
- A course recently attended where an update on health and safety was given
- A new way of dismantling sharps that reduces the risk of an injury

In addition, you may want to ask your patients for their opinions and suggestions. However, be mindful of how you approach this as you do not want to raise concerns unnecessarily.

Collate the information received, match it with your initial study and put it in an order of priority. The **MOP** approach is quite useful:

- Must address immediately before anything else
- Ought to address within a set timescale
- Prefer to address now but other issues will take priority

Once you have done this you can now refer to the manual. Select the relevant chapters from your MOP list and determine if you are doing enough or if not, what can be done to improve the situation and how are you going to achieve it?

Remember, you do not have to read this manual all at once; it might be better to set reasonable targets and plan your schedule. Utilise the skills and knowledge within your team effectively to help develop your health and safety systems and procedures.

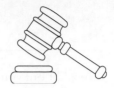

Introduction – legal information

Scope of this chapter

- Introduction
- Statute and common law
- Non-legislative guidance
- Law enforcement
- The Health and Safety at Work etc. Act 1974
- European Regulations
- Legislation update

Introduction

When it comes to health and safety, you may be wondering what all the fuss is about. Let us face it, we are health-care professionals and more specifically dental professionals. Therefore, we genuinely care about the health, safety, welfare and well-being of people. We demonstrate this on a daily basis by providing quality service which is people centred and where risks are effectively managed. However, the Health and Safety Executive (HSE) work-related accident statistics for 2007–2008 show that employers have neglected their responsibility to protect employees and that accidents have occurred. This not only has an effect on the injured party and his/her family but also on the business, where the absence of an employee can severely disrupt business operations. Keeping this in the context of what we are

actually dealing with, it has been said that dental settings are relatively low-risk environments and consist of predominantly 'non-complex' risks. With this in mind, a simple and straightforward approach to managing health and safety, which involves every member of the team, is therefore more appropriate. It is important for individuals to have an understanding of health and safety law, what their responsibilities are and how to apply the law to everything they do. In this section, we will address the key aspects of health and safety legislation, providing a comprehensive overview but keeping it concise.

Statute and common law

The law regarding health and safety is a combination of criminal law set out in 'Statutes' that deals with crimes against the State and common law which settles disputes between individuals or organisations.

Statute law

Statute law is the written law of the land and consists of Acts of Parliament and the associated Statutory Instruments, for example, rules, regulations or orders which are made within the parameters of the Acts. The purpose of statute law is to deal with 'wrong doings' committed against society as a whole and to act as a deterrent for repetition. Punishment for 'wrong doings' for those who are found guilty, 'beyond all reasonable doubt' (BARD) is determined by the judges and could result in a maximum fine and/or imprisonment.

Breaches of statute law can be used in civil claims where there is a need to establish negligence. However, this may not be possible if such a breach is prohibited by the particular Act of Parliament or Regulation.

Types of statutory duties

There are four types of statutory duties which allow different responses to duties imposed upon individuals and the wording of a statutory duty is most significant as it sets out the legal standard that must be achieved.

1. **Absolute duty** – the words 'must' or 'shall' are used, which emphasise that the duty is imposed. It has been determined that certain steps must be taken to control the hazard; therefore, these are compulsory and the duty holder has no choice.
2. **Practicable** – the words 'so far as is practicable' will appear, which allow the duty holder to consider whether it is physically possible to take such control measures in the light of current technology, cost and feasibility. In this situation, the employer can apply a degree of reason to the situation.
3. **Reasonably practicable** – the words 'so far as is reasonably practicable' are used which allow the duty holder to balance the cost of taking such action against the risk presented. If the cost is seen to far outweigh the risk, then steps do not need to be taken. Caution must be taken to ensure all eventualities have been analysed and the employer can prove that the steps taken are the best under the circumstances.
4. **Reasonable care** – the words 'to take reasonable care' are used, which require the duty holder to consider the effects of action or inaction. If the consequences of action or inaction are reasonably foreseeable there is a requirement to avoid the negative outcome.

Common law

Common law has evolved over time as a result of previous cases and decisions made in courts by judges. The common law cases have resulted in setting down principles which act as precedents and help determine the outcome in future cases. The purpose of an action taken in a civil court is to recognise the loss or damage suffered, to restore the injured party to the state they were in before the accident happened by financial means and to compensate for the pain or suffering. A civil claim for compensation may be reduced if it is proven that the injured party has contributed to the injury or ill health suffered – for example, by failing to wear personal protective equipment or not following a safe working procedure. This is known as *contributory negligence*. Civil actions have to be started within 3 years of the accident happening or the injury being recognised. In a number of cases, civil claims are resolved before they get to court by an agreed sum of money being paid to the injured party and therefore the case is settled out of court. If agreement cannot be reached then the case is taken to court but both parties need to be aware that court costs have to be settled and these may be high.

Non-legislative guidance

As previously mentioned, health and safety law consists of Acts of Parliament, Regulations and associated Statutory Instruments. This section will provide an overview of the additional sources of information that do not have the same legal status as Acts or Regulations but should be used by duty holders. It should be mentioned that these **could** have quasi-legal status (almost legal) in a court of law and therefore may be used to influence the outcome if the guidance has not been followed.

- Approved Codes of Practice (ACOPs) – authorised by Parliament to provide practical guidance on how to comply with Acts and Regulations. Failure to comply with an ACOP **could** render the duty holder liable for offence.

- Guidance Notes – issued by the HSE to provide advice, guidance and suggestions on how to comply with Acts and Regulations; they demonstrate what is deemed to be best practice. They have no legal standing but **could** be used to determine aspects of prosecutions.
- British Standards – indicates best practice within a specific aspect of health and safety. Some British Standards are approved by HSE and therefore have the same legal status as ACOPs.

In addition to the above, occupational specific professional guidance should also be used which is designed to provide best practice.

Law enforcement

The responsibility for enforcing health and safety law is split between the following authorities/agencies:

- Health and Safety Executive (HSE) – is responsible for factories, schools, hospitals, doctors and dental practices. Enforced by HSE inspectors
- Local Authority – is responsible for retail outlets, warehousing, hotel and catering, restaurants, sports and leisure facilities. Enforced by Environmental Health Officers (EHOs)
- Fire Authority – is responsible for fire safety regulations in all workplaces. Enforced by the local fire brigade (Exceptions exist, e.g. construction sites.)
- Police Force – is responsible for investigating cases relating to Corporate Manslaughter (England, Wales and Northern Ireland) and Corporate Homicide (Scotland) Act 2007

Please note that the above-mentioned responsibilities are intended to provide guidance only. In premises where a range of activities are undertaken, it is the primary activity that determines the enforcing authority.

Powers of inspectors

The powers of inspectors are wide ranging and range from routine inspections of premises to investigations following an accident or complaint. The frequency of routine inspections is often determined by the risk levels in a particular workplace. Therefore, it could be said that factory premises are a higher risk than dental practices. Employers should fully cooperate with all aspects of the inspection before, during and after. This could include request for information, presence of personnel, access to documents and an action plan for areas of improvement. Listed below are some of the powers:

- Entering at all reasonable times (if an accident has happened or a complaint has been made inspectors may enter at any time)
- Carrying out investigations
- Employing the police, if necessary, to assist with investigations
- Dismantling and removing equipment
- Taking measurements, samples, products, articles and photographs
- Inspecting, seizing or copying documents
- Interviewing personnel and asking questions
- Seizing a substance or article and destroying it or making it safe
- Anything else necessary in the light of the investigation
- Taking appropriate **action** in light of the findings

Actions available to inspectors

The outcome of an inspection and the subsequent actions will depend upon the findings and can include the following:

- Verbal advice and recommendations on how to improve and develop. This should be adhered to and implemented.
- Written advice stating what must be done to rectify the situation and the reasons for such action. Advice in writing will normally constitute a formal warning and the duty holder will need to confirm that rectifications have been carried out.

If there is a breach of an Act or Regulation then a legal notice can be issued. This could be as follows:

- An Improvement notice specifying what the breach is and when it must be rectified. The duty holder has 21 days to appeal against the notice, during which time the notice is suspended.
- A Prohibition notice is issued when there is a serious risk of personal injury. This prohibits the particular activity from being undertaken, usually with immediate effect, until further action is taken. The duty holder can appeal but the notice remains in effect and therefore is not suspended during that period.
- A Prosecution may be brought against a company or an individual in certain circumstances – for example, if the breach has resulted in death, disregard for health and safety requirements or failure to comply with a legal notice.

Additional information

Section 10 of The Health and Safety at Work etc. Act 1974 established two bodies to carry out health and safety functions on behalf of the Crown. The two bodies were known as the Health and Safety Commission (HSC) responsible for developing policies and the Health and Safety Executive (HSE) responsible for advice and enforcement. In 2008, these two bodies merged, bringing together their powers and functions, and the name Health and Safety Executive has been retained.

The Health and Safety at Work etc. Act 1974

The Health and Safety at Work etc. Act 1974 is the primary piece of legislation on Health and Safety in Great Britain. The principle of the Act is to ensure the health, safety and welfare of those at work and others who may be affected by that work. It achieves this by placing broad general duties on the following people:

- Employers
  They have a common law duty to take reasonable care of employees. Employers must, so far as is reasonably practicable, safeguard

the health, safety and welfare of employees by providing and maintaining
  - safe equipment and systems to work safely;
  - safe handling, storage and transport of items and substances;
  - information, instruction, training and supervision;
  - safe workplace, with safe access to and egress from;
  - safe working environment with adequate and appropriate welfare facilities.
  An employer must
  - prepare a written statement of general Health and Safety Policy (where five or more employed);
  - set out the organisation and arrangements for carrying out the policy;
  - review, revise and bring to the attention of employees the safety policy;
  - consult with employees on health and safety issues;
  - provide safety equipment and clothing free of charge;
  - consult with safety representatives and safety committees where applicable.

In addition to the above, employers have a duty so far as is reasonably practicable, to other persons not employed – for example, members of the public or service engineers.

- Employees
  This includes all employees including managers and supervisors and everyone who has a contract of employment.
  Employees must
  - take reasonable care of their own health and safety;
  - take reasonable care for the health and safety of others who may be affected by their actions or inactions;
  - cooperate with the employer to enable the employer to meet his/her legal duties;
  - not intentionally interfere or misuse anything provided in the interests of health, safety or welfare.
- Self-employed
  The duties are as for employers with the exception of the safety policy, unless they

employ people. In addition, they should take steps

- ☐ to ensure their own health and safety;
- ☐ to ensure the health and safety of others who may be affected by their actions.

■ Those in control of premises

Specific responsibilities are listed below; however, in the situation where landlords or managing agents are involved, responsibilities for 'control' will be detailed in the tenancy agreement.

They should

- ☐ ensure that premises are safe without risks to health;
- ☐ ensure safe access to and egress from premises;
- ☐ maintain and repair premises;
- ☐ ensure that equipment or substances provided are, so far as is reasonably practicable, safe and without risks to health.

■ Designers, manufacturers, suppliers and importers

The duty holders must ensure that articles (objects) and substances are safe when being used; in particular,

- ☐ articles are designed with safety in mind, tested and examined and bear the appropriate safety standard marking;
- ☐ adequate information is provided about the safe use and any revisions subsequently provided;
- ☐ equipment is installed safely and duty holders must ensure it can be used safely after installation.

Offences and penalties

Successful prosecutions under the Act carry a maximum fine of £20,000 in a Magistrates Court, with an unlimited fine in the Crown Court and up to 2 years imprisonment for certain offences. For a criminal prosecution to be successful, the courts must prove 'beyond all reasonable doubt' (BARD) that the employer failed to demonstrate reasonableness and the injuries sustained were a direct result of this failure.

In summary, the Health and Safety at Work etc. Act 1974 covers everyone involved with work or affected by it. It is built on general duties to cover all possible hazards and is designed to encourage employers to improve standards and performance. It creates a framework for developing and updating health and safety law and hence it is known as an *enabling Act*.

European Regulations

In 1993, more specific regulations were introduced to cover all the risks connected with health and safety at work. The aim of the regulations was to guarantee an improved level of protection for people at work and to ensure that all members of the European Union adopted a 'standardised' approach to the management of health and safety. The 1993 Regulations were commonly termed the 'Six Pack' and consisted of six sets of regulations which addressed the need to

- ■ manage health and safety including assessing and controlling risks;
- ■ ensure the safety of the workplace including the structure and its facilities;
- ■ provide and maintain safe equipment and systems of working;
- ■ conduct the operation and use of display screen equipment safely and assess the associated risks;
- ■ assess the moving and handling of objects to determine the need for such an activity and eliminate or reduce risks;
- ■ provide suitable and appropriate personal protection as a last resort where risks cannot be suitably controlled by other means.

Since 1993, a range of other regulations have come into force and are detailed throughout this manual. It is important for employers to comply with the regulations but they do not have to provide all the facilities mentioned, provided they can ensure, so far as is reasonably practicable, the health, safety, welfare and well-being of employees and others affected.

Legislation update

Source: Hammonds Safety Health and Environment Group.

The Corporate Manslaughter (England, Wales and Northern Ireland) and Corporate Homicide

(Scotland) Act 2007 will allow the prosecution of companies for the death of an individual. The organisation will be guilty of an offence if the way they managed or organised their activities

- causes a person's death;
- amounts to gross breach of a relevant duty of care owed by the organisation (employer) to the deceased.

An organisation is guilty of an offence, only if the ways in which its activities are managed or organised by the person/s who play a significant role in making decisions about the way activities are undertaken are negligent. The introduction of the Act places an even greater emphasis on people understanding their specific responsibilities for health and safety and ensuring that they have the knowledge and skill to carry them out.

Summary

Acts of Parliament, Regulations and the associated non-legislative guidance set out minimum standards which employers are required to comply. Throughout this manual you will find a combination of all the above. Compare these with your own organisational standards and identify where improvements need to be made in order to demonstrate compliance and ensure the health, safety, welfare and well-being of people.

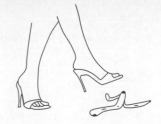

1 Accidents and first aid

Scope of this chapter

- Introduction
- Legislation
- Accidents
- Nature, causes and prevention
- Reporting and recording
- Investigating
- Insurance
- First aid
- Purpose
- First aid provision
- Training

Figures

Figure 1.1 – Accident report form.
Figure 1.2 – Significant event analysis report.

Introduction

The primary aim of this manual is to assist those working in dental environments to manage health and safety by assessing risks and implementing reasonable control measures which are aimed at preventing accidents and cases of ill health. It is generally considered that dental settings, in particular, general dental practices, are relatively low-risk environments if we compare them with other industry sectors such as construction sites or factories. However, a proactive approach to accident prevention is vital for the following reasons:

- Ethical – employers have a moral duty of care to protect employees and others.
- Legal – employers and employees must demonstrate compliance with legislation.
- Organisational – health and safety policies and procedures should be a condition of employment.
- Financial – it makes economic sense to reduce workdays lost from accidents and ill health.

The cost of workplace accidents can have a detrimental effect on the business as well as on the injured party and their immediate family. In order to successfully prevent accidents everyone must first have an understanding of how they are caused, the accident types and what procedure to follow if an accident happens.

Managing Health and Safety in the Dental Practice: A Practical Guide, by Jane Bonehill   © 2010 by Blackwell Publishing Ltd.

Legislation

- Health and Safety at Work etc. Act 1974:

  Employers shall ensure, so far as is reasonably practicable, the health, safety and welfare at work of their employees and anyone else who may be affected by their business activities in order to prevent accidents.

- Management of Health and Safety at Work Regulations 1999:

  Employers must undertake suitable and sufficient assessments of risks to the health and safety of employees and implement reasonable controls in order to prevent accidents. Investigating the causes of accidents is an essential part of good health and safety management and assists with reviewing risk assessments.

- Reporting of Injuries, Diseases and Dangerous Occurrences Regulations 1995 (RIDDOR):

  Employers are required to report certain specified accidents and dangerous occurrences to the enforcing authority, via the HSE's incident contact centre, if they arise out of or in connection with work activities.

- Health and Safety (First Aid) Regulations 1981:

  Employers should make an assessment of first-aid needs appropriate to the circumstances of the workplace and make available equipment and facilities enabling first-aid to be rendered.

- The Social Security (Claims and Payments) Amendment (No 2) Regulations 2006:

  Employers are required to investigate the circumstances of every accident that is reported and record the circumstances if there is a discrepancy between what was initially reported and the investigation findings.

- Employers' Liability (Compulsory Insurance) Regulations 1998:

  Employers must have sufficient insurance which ensures that if employees are injured or made ill at work they are able to make a civil claim against their employer.

Accidents

The latest accident statistics (2007–2008) produced by the Health and Safety Executive (HSE) show that there has been a reduction in workplace accidents. This could be as a result of employers communicating health and safety more effectively, so that employees are more safety conscious or because under-reporting exists. Under-reporting is a factor that must be considered when relying on statistics to inform us on health and safety at work. In this chapter, we will address the range of requirements to report workplace accidents in order to ensure that statistics provide reliable information.

Nature, causes and prevention

Nature

It is important to understand what the term *accident* actually means as there are a number of variations. The most common definition is 'an unplanned, uncontrolled event which has the **potential** to cause injury'. The word *potential* is vitally important in the definition as it helps us to appreciate that not all accidents result in injury. However, all accidents need to be addressed as part of accident prevention. Accidents are sometimes divided into five categories as follows:

1. Death or major injury – reportable to enforcing authority
2. Over 3-day injury – reportable to enforcing authority
3. Minor injury – not reportable to enforcing authority
4. Dangerous occurrence – no injury but reportable to enforcing authority
5. Near miss – no injury, not reportable to enforcing authority if it does not fall under categories 1, 2 and 4

The above-mentioned categories link to accident reporting, which will be addressed later in this chapter. As you will notice from the above categories, not all accidents result in injury. However, today's accident, if it recurs, has the potential to cause injury tomorrow if not addressed.

Causes

Accidents do not just happen. There are underlying causative factors that bring about the situation in the first place. It may not be possible to prevent all accidents but if we have a general understanding of what can cause them to happen we are better equipped to implement accident prevention measures. Accidents are usually caused by the following four factors.

- Human – people behave unsafely or forget to do something; unsafe acts or omissions.
- Occupational – relating to dentistry; for example, we are exposed to harmful substances, we use hazardous equipment and some activities are potentially risky.
- Environmental – workplace conditions could pose a risk, for example, extremes of temperature or poor housekeeping.
- Organisational – health and safety is not managed effectively or efficiently.

Accidents do not usually happen as a result of one factor. They occur as a result of a chain of events. This chain of events is illustrated in the following list of possible causes of accidents that take the above four factors to the next level of understanding.

- **Management control** – management systems, policies and procedures are inappropriate or out of date, or delegation is ineffective.
- **Health and safety culture** – the organisation permits risk taking; there is a lack of health and safety training or no system of communicating information.
- **Unsafe acts/unsafe conditions** – unsafe equipment or substances, unsafe systems of work which create unsafe working practices.
- **Accidents** – that go unrecognised or unreported and are therefore not investigated.

- **Injuries** – resulting in various types of injuries from minor to severe.

As you can see from the above illustration there is a chain of events that has a knock-on effect resulting in an accident. The causative factors have the potential to result in a range of accident types from the most severe which result in death or major injury to the less severe which result in minor injury or no injury. It is usually the less severe that go unreported. However, these can provide valuable information in accident prevention as they help to reduce the risk of something more serious occurring.

Prevention

All chapters within this manual are aimed at preventing accidents and include the physical workplace, work equipment, hazardous substances, management systems and working practices. The list below specifically addresses the causative factors mentioned earlier.

- **Management control** – appropriately designed health and safety policy which reflects the needs of the organisation clearly shows lines of responsibility and accountability and has adequate arrangements in place. Policy is consulted on and communicated, reviewed at planned intervals and revised as necessary.
- **Health and safety culture** – everyone is committed to making the policy work, capabilities are assessed and training needs identified and there exists an open communication process where people speak freely about concerns and comments.
- **Unsafe acts/unsafe conditions** – systems are in place which identify and assess hazardous situations, controls are implemented before something goes wrong and safe operating procedures exist for all at-risk activities.
- **Accidents** – all accidents are reported, recorded and investigated, including near misses.
- **Injuries** – the more severe injuries are reduced and appropriate first aid is provided based on an assessment of need.

Evidence shows that there are more near-miss accidents than those that result in major injury. In order to reduce the risk of the near misses moving up the scale to something more serious, it is important to report and record each and every accident that happens.

Reporting and recording

Accident reporting and recording is essential in order to meet organisational and legislative requirements. Specific reasons are as follows:

Organisational
- Identify the underlying causes and implement preventive measures.
- Prevent a similar occurrence.
- Identify patterns and trends which could indicate a failure in the management systems.
- Demonstrate compliance with the policy for reporting and recording if there is a litigation claim.

Legislative
- Comply with legal requirements for certain types of accidents (see section Reporting procedures).
- Reporting provides national statistics to enforcement agencies in order to issue guidance, revise legislation and target resources more effectively.

Reporting procedures

All organisations, regardless of the size, should have a responsible person for employees to report to if an accident occurs. This person will be named in Part 2 of the Health and Safety Policy. The named person will then record the particulars of the accident, ensuring that sufficient detail is obtained; Figure 1.1 provides an example of what is meant by sufficient detail. This form also complies with The Social Security (Claims and Payments) Amendment Regulations 2006 which requires employers, where 10 or more people are employed, to record all accidents at work. Alternatively, employers may choose to use the

Accident Book B1510 obtained from HSE. The named person will then determine if there is a legal requirement to report to the enforcing authority under Reporting of Injuries, Diseases and Dangerous Occurrences Regulations 1995 (RIDDOR).

Reporting under RIDDOR

Any of the following arising out of, or in connection with, work activities must be reported to the Incident Contact Centre (ICC) or the local HSE. The reporting procedures vary according to the type of accident/incident; however, in all cases this should be done as soon as possible using Form F2508 for injuries or F2508A for diseases. Reporting can be done by telephone, online, email or post (See Sources of advice and information on page 256).

Notify ICC or HSE immediately by telephone and complete form F2508 within 10 days in the event of the following:

- Death of an employee or self-employed person working on the premises
- Death suffered by a member of the public or if he/she is taken to hospital for treatment
- A major injury (including as a result of physical violence) suffered by an employee or self-employed person working on your premises or working in somebody else's premises (see section Reportable major injuries)
- A dangerous occurrence that has taken place (see section Reportable dangerous occurrences)
- A reportable disease that has been diagnosed by a medical practitioner (Form F2508A see section Reportable diseases)

Notify ICC or HSE in writing; complete form F2508 within 10 days in the event of the following:

- An employee or self-employed is absent from work or unable to do his/her normal work for more than three consecutive days.

Three consecutive days is not counting the day of the accident but including non-worked days. This means that rest days must be included.

Figure 1.1 Accident report form.

A. The accident report form contains personal details that must be kept confidential in compliance with the Data Protection Act. After completion, **Part B** must be passed to the person responsible for record storage and kept for a period of at least 3 years from the date the accident happened.

Name of person who had the accident . . . . Accident No: . . . .

✂ . . . .

B.1. Who is completing this form? (please circle)   (A). Person who had the accident   (B). Someone else (please record details below)

Name: . . . .

Address . . . . ,,,

. . . . ,,,,, ... Tel number . . . .

Relationship/Association to the person who had the accident . . . .

2. Person who had the accident (please circle)   Employee/Self-employed   Visitor   Patient   Other(please specify) . . . .

Name . . . .

Home address . . . .

. . . . Tel no . . . .

Occupation . . . .

3. When did the accident happen: dd/mm/yy . . . .

4. Where did the accident happen (exact location) . . . .

5. What circumstances lead to the accident happening? . . . .

. . . . ,,,,,, ... ||||| . . . .

. . . .

6. What were the consequences of the accident, e.g. injury, disease, ill health, time lost by casualty? . . . .

. . . .

7. Was any first aid treatment administered? (please circle)   YES (If yes please complete sections below)   NO

Treatment administered . . . .

Who administered treatment & their position . . . .

8. What happened to the casualty following the accident, e.g. sent home, referred to hospital etc? . . . .

9. The person completing this accident report form and the casualty (if these are different) must sign and date in the spaces provided.

The information contained in this document is a true and accurate account of the accident.

a. SIGNATURE: Person completing the accident record form . . . .

b. SIGNATURE: Person who had the accident . . . .

10. Is this accident reportable under RIDDOR?(please circle)   YES   NO

Date reported to the enforcing authority & RIDDOR Reference Number . . . .

Name & position of person reporting to enforcing authority . . . .

Notify ICC or HSE within 1 year in writing in the event of the following:

- Death of an employee within 1 year of the date of an accident as a result of a reportable injury or condition at work (even if it had been previously reported).

Reportable major injuries are as follows:

- Fracture of a bone, other than fingers, thumbs or toes
- Amputation
- Dislocation of the shoulder, hip, knee or spine
- Loss of sight (temporary or permanent)
- Chemical or hot metal burn to the eye or any penetrating injury to the eye
- Injury resulting from an electric shock or electrical burn leading to unconsciousness or requiring resuscitation or admittance to hospital for more than 24 hours
- Any other injury leading to hypothermia, heat-induced illness or unconsciousness or requiring resuscitation or admittance to hospital for more than 24 hours
- Unconsciousness caused by asphyxia or exposure to a harmful substance or biological agent
- Acute illness requiring medical treatment or loss of consciousness arising from absorption of any substance by inhalation, ingestion or through the skin
- Acute illness requiring medical treatment where there is reason to believe that this resulted from exposure to a biological agent or its toxins or infected material

The potential exists for all of the above to happen in dental settings, although some are highly unlikely.

Reportable dangerous occurrences are as follows (only those relevant to dental settings listed):

- Collapse, overturning or failure of lifting equipment such as hoists
- Failure of a pressure vessel where the failure had the potential to cause death
- Electric short circuit or overload causing fire or explosion

- Accidental release of a biological agent likely to cause human illness
- Failure of radiation equipment to return to its safe position after exposure period
- Collapse of scaffolding over 5 m high (construction work being undertaken)
- A dangerous substance being transported by road involved in a fire or released (substantial quantities need to be involved; this may apply to travelling on domiciliary visits)
- Unintended collapse of a building or its structures during alteration or demolition where more than 5 tonnes of material falls (construction work being undertaken)
- Any explosion or fire causing suspension of work for more than 24 hours
- Sudden uncontrolled release of flammable liquid or gas (quantities apply)
- Accidental release of any substance which might damage health

Reportable diseases are as follows (only those relevant to dental settings listed):

- Disease of the skin, bones or blood due to ionising radiation
- Cramp of the hand or forearm due to repetitive movements (typing or handwriting)
- Traumatic inflammation of the tendons of the hand or forearm (constrained postures or extremes or flexion of the hand or wrist)
- Carpal tunnel syndrome (use of hand-held vibrating tools)
- Hand–arm vibration syndrome (use of hand-held rotary tools in grinding, sanding or polishing)
- Hepatitis (contact with human blood or blood products)
- Tuberculosis (exposure to a person who might be the source of infection)
- Occupational dermatitis (skin contact with certain sensitising material, e.g. latex)
- Occupational asthma (exposure through inhalation to certain sensitising material such as chemicals)

For other reportable dangerous occurrences and reportable diseases please refer HSE Website A-Z Index R.

The accident report/record must be kept at the workplace for a period of 3 years from the date of the accident or the report/record being made. The storage of accident report/record forms must comply with the Data Protection Act and be held in a secure medium that is not accessible to unauthorised persons for the purpose of maintaining the confidentiality of personal information. Secure medium may include a locked filing cabinet or password-protected electronic system.

Investigating

There is no precise duty in health and safety law to investigate workplace accidents, but this is implied in various regulations. For example, the Management of Health and Safety at Work Regulations 1999 considers accident investigation to be an integral part of any management system and helps to inform the risk assessment review process. In addition, The Social Security (Claims and Payments) Amendment Regulations 2006 requires employers to take reasonable steps to investigate accidents and to record the circumstances as this may have to be disclosed at a later date. In addition to the legal considerations, accident investigation is an essential element of accident prevention. The accident should be investigated as soon as possible after the event while it is still fresh in everyone's mind. It should be coordinated by a competent person and involve all necessary people. There are different levels of investigation ranging from that which is suitable for potentially less serious accidents which can be investigated using a 'significant event analysis', to an in-depth and complex investigative technique for accidents where the consequences have the potential to be more serious. Whichever level is most appropriate the investigation should include the following:

- The gathering of information
- An analysis of information
- The selection of suitable control or preventive measures
- An action plan with timed implementation based on priority

Significant event analysis

Significant event analysis (Figure 1.2) is a key requirement of clinical governance as part of the Department of Health National Health Service (NHS) improvement plan. Significant event analysis is contained within the *Standards for Better Health*. All those providing dentistry must have this in place in order to protect patients. A significant event includes anything that has happened and had the potential to affect the safety of patients. The analysis is a useful discipline to apply in the event of an accident investigation. It should include the following:

- Identification of the exact location where it took place
- The nature of the event, clinical or non-clinical
- People involved in the event
- A description of the event and whether any injury was sustained or any other outcome was recognised
- An analysis of the causative factors which contributed to the event happening
- The arrival at a decision as to whether the event could have been prevented and an explanation for the decision
- Any other significant matters that need to be reported, that is, legally required to be reported under RIDDOR
- Corrective actions required to prevent recurrence and priority given
- A check to see that action has been taken and its effectiveness

Significant event analysis should be shared with other dental professionals in order to learn from them and improve patient safety. The reporting forms should be returned to the appropriate body [Primary Care Trust (PCT) or Deanery] annually where they will be used as a resource for fellow practitioners.

Complex accident investigation

Where the consequences are potentially more serious it may be necessary to carry out the

Figure 1.2   Significant event analysis report.

Exact location of the significant event	
Clinical or non-clinical	Persons involved
Describe the event that took place, any injury sustained or outcome.	
What factors appear to have contributed to the event?	
Could the event have been prevented? YES NO (please circle) Describe the reason for your answer:	
Are there any other matters you need to report?	
What corrective actions are to be taken to prevent recurrence and when will they be implemented?	
Corrective action implemented (please specify date)	
Person completing this report	Date

following procedure to obtain information: this builds on information obtained in the previously mentioned accident report form (Figure 1.1).

- A description of the accident as reported
- The circumstances which appear to have led to it happening and any contributory factors
- The consequences of the accident, for example, injury, disease and near miss
- Whether any first aid was given
- The potential for the accident to happen again and the harm that may occur
- Whether the accident was related to a task where a risk assessment had been undertaken and if the control measures were adequate
- The competence of those involved, training received and supervision arrangements
- Any previous occurrences
- Determining who will be interviewed and their need for a representative
- Any other supporting documents required, that is, training records, previous accident records, first aid log, risk assessments, hazard report forms, equipment maintenance records, etc.
- Preparation of open questions to assist in identifying causative factors. This should include factors relating to the premises, equipment, substances, working practices, competency of people and management systems such as risk assessments
- Involving the interviewees in finding solutions to preventing recurrences
- Inspecting the scene of the accident, studying all relevant aspects and carrying out appropriate research
- Involving others both internally and externally and seeking advice from others such as defence organisation or insurance company
- Determining if there has been a breach of legislation or organisational policy
- Formulating a report of your findings and recommendations
- Taking action to prevent recurrence
- Monitoring actions to check whether they are effective and rectifying if necessary

The findings of the above may require risk assessments and safe operating procedures to be reviewed and revised.

Insurance

Employers are legally required to have employers' liability insurance. This is designed to ensure that if employees are injured or made ill at work they can make a civil claim against their employers. The insurance cover must be sufficient to pay any damages awarded to the injured party. Damages are awarded in civil courts. Failure to comply with the legislation, however, is a criminal offence and can result in severe fines every day without appropriate cover. In October 2008, the requirement to display the certificate of insurance was amended and businesses can now 'display' the certificate electronically, provided it can be made readily available to employees and enforcement officers. Certificates must be retained for a period of 40 years after the last date on which they were valid. Public liability insurance is not a compulsory requirement in law. However, dental practices will find it worthwhile to have this type of insurance cover because of the nature of the business. For example, a claim could be made by a member of the public or a patient.

First aid

Employees can become ill or suffer injuries during the course of their work. It is important that they receive attention immediately to prevent injuries from becoming worse. It must be recognised that first aid is the initial management of injury or ill health. All employers have a responsibility to make available adequate and appropriate first aid arrangements, equipment and facilities. The employer must inform the employees about the first aid arrangements, including the location of equipment and facilities and the person responsible for first aid.

Purpose

The overall purpose of first aid is to provide treatment to employees for minor injuries which do not require further treatment by a medical practitioner. Or to provide immediate assistance to prevent situations from becoming worse and therefore to preserve life while waiting for medical help to arrive.

First aid provision

In order to determine what first aid equipment and facilities are required, an assessment of need must be carried out. The assessment should consider the following:

- Hazards currently present and extent of the risks
- Control measures in place to reduce risks
- Size of the practice, number of people employed and present at any one time
- Individual competencies of employees
- Accident history and statistics, any patterns and trends identified
- Systems in place to manage health and safety
- The need for additional facilities in the case of lone workers
- Exceptional circumstances which could increase, for example, if construction work is taking place

A range of equipment and facilities is available to choose from.

First aid box

Minimum contents of a first aid box include the following:

- General guidance leaflet
- Twenty individually wrapped sterile adhesive dressings
- Two sterile eye pads
- Four individually wrapped sterile triangular bandages
- Six safety pins
- Six medium and two large-sized individually wrapped sterile unmedicated wound dressings
- One pair of disposable gloves

First aid boxes must not contain any medicinal products such as tablets, inhalers, ointments or creams. If the assessment of need identifies that eye wash is required then this should be located at a designated eye wash station. First aid boxes must be clearly identified by a green background with a white St. George's cross, and the location communicated to employees. More than one box may be needed to ensure that adequate facilities are provided according to the number of people employed at any one time. Boxes must be checked regularly to ensure that contents are not out of date and are replaced after use.

Travelling first aid kits

For dental professionals who provide regular and routine domiciliary care for patients, there may be the need for such a kit. The minimum contents of the kit should be as described earlier.

First aid room

This facility is usually required in large organisations or where complex risks exist. The room should be readily accessible, clearly signposted, contain appropriate facilities and equipment and be used solely for the purpose of first aid. It is unlikely that this will be needed in a general dental practice.

First aid personnel

An adequate and appropriate number of first aid personnel must be provided. The number is determined by the results of the earlier assessment. Table 1.1 gives guidance on the provision of first aid personnel.

Appointed person

This is the minimum level of personnel that an employer has to provide. Appointed persons are not fully qualified first aiders and therefore do not have the same responsibilities; they are appointed

Table 1.1 Guidance on the provision of first aid personnel.

Category of risk	Number of employees at any location	Suggested number of first aid personnel
Lower risk – shops, offices and dental practices	Fewer than 50	At least one appointed person
	50–100 (e.g. dental hospitals)	At least one first aider
Medium risk – light engineering, e.g. dental laboratories	Fewer than 20	At least one appointed person
	20–100	At least one first aider for every 50 employed
Higher risk – construction, chemical manufacture	Fewer than 5	At least one appointed person
	5–50	At least one first aider

Source: HSE.

to take charge when someone is injured or falls ill. This includes calling an ambulance if needed, restocking the first aid box/kit and, if necessary, dealing with minor wound bleeding. From Table 1.1 you may have determined that this level of provision is adequate for general dental practices, but you may also need to appoint more than one person in the event of absences. Appointed persons should be competent to carry out their responsibilities and therefore will require at least a minimum level of training.

First aiders

If the assessment of need identifies that this level of personnel is required employers must ensure the person is capable and competent to carry out their responsibility. They should be sufficient in number and absences should be considered. When selecting first aiders, employers will need to consider the following attributes such as reliability, ability to remain calm in an emergency, effective communication skills and the ability to learn new skills and absorb knowledge and be able to cope with the demands of an emergency situation. First aiders must be trained in administering first aid. Training has to have been approved by HSE and individuals must hold a current certificate.

Training

Before carrying out either of the above roles the person must undergo training to equip himself/herself with the skills and knowledge required to carry out the role effectively and competently.

Appointed person

There is no regulatory requirement to provide training for appointed persons. However, employers should consider the need for basic first aid training in order for the individuals to carry out their role as described earlier. In addition, employers may decide to send the persons on the new 1-day emergency first aid at work (EFAW) course approved by HSE from 1 October 2009, which will enable them to become first aiders in regulatory terms.

First aiders

First aiders must hold a valid certificate of competence. As from 1 October 2009, the HSE-approved course for first aid in the workplace will become the 3-day First Aid at Work (FAW) course. First aid training must be renewed every 3 years as decided by the HSE (correct at the time of writing). This is because the certificate of competence expires every 3 years. Employers should keep records of training and arrange for refresher training and retesting before the certificate expires. If the certificate expires the individual will have to undertake a full course of training to be re-established as a first aider.

Summary

In dental settings, we may not have to deal with the more serious accidents because of the nature of dentistry, being relatively low risk. However, accidents can happen and these must be reported, recorded, investigated and acted upon in order to prevent an escalation of the situation to something more serious or a recurrence of the accident. First aid can assist in preventing the effects of injuries from becoming worse and can aid recovery.

Action – check the following

- Do you have a reliable accident reporting procedure?
- Does your reporting procedure include an investigation or analysis of the event that took place?
- Does your investigation or analysis help to prevent accidents?
- Do you have adequate and appropriate first aid provision to meet your needs?

Frequently asked questions

Q. If a self-employed person, for example, a hygienist, has a RIDDOR reportable accident, who is responsible for reporting this?
A. The responsibility lies with the occupier of the premises. This will be the owner or the person with whom the hygienist has the contract.
Q. How do we calculate an over-3-day injury?
A. The day the accident happened is not included in the calculation; however, any non-work days such as rest days, are included. For example, if the person has the accident on Thursday, then Friday is day 1 of the calculation. If Saturday and Sunday are rest days these count as days 2 and 3, if the person does not return to work on Monday this is day 4; therefore, this is an over-3-day injury.
Q. Should we investigate all accidents including near misses?
A. Near misses are accidents which do not result in an injury; however, they need to be investigated to examine the underlying causes. For example, it may be identified that the event happened because of a lack of training. This factor will still exist and, therefore, has the potential to cause injury next time.
Q. Are dental practices legally required to employ a trained and qualified first aider on the premises?
A. How much first aid provision is dependent upon the circumstances in the individual practice? An assessment of need is required, taking into consideration the risk levels present, which will help determine if a qualified first aider is needed. The assessment may identify that there is no need for a qualified first aider and therefore an appointed person is adequate and appropriate.
Q. Do we have to provide first aid equipment and facilities for our patients?
A. The regulations require employers to make the provision for employees, not for non-employees. However, a duty of care exists to people other than employees; therefore, the provision should be extended for patients.

Links to other chapters

Chapter 11 – Lone working
Chapter 12 – Managing health and safety
Chapter 14 – Medical emergencies
Chapter 19 – Risk assessment

2 Alcohol, drugs and smoking

Scope of this chapter

- Introduction
- Legislation
- Principles of working safely
- The effects of alcohol, drugs and smoking
- The smoke-free workplace
- Managing alcohol and drug abuse
- Professional implications of alcohol and drug abuse

Figures

Figure 2.1 – Model alcohol and drugs policy.

Introduction

When drugs are referred to in this chapter it is the use of controlled substances and the misuse of over-the-counter or prescription drugs which is meant. Controlled substances include class A, B and C drugs such as cannabis, cocaine, lysergic acid diethylamide (LSD), etc. The term 'drugs' is also used to include the abuse of other substances such as solvent abuse. The use of such drugs is illegal and it may seem surprising that this chapter also includes alcohol and smoking when alcohol and tobacco are not in themselves illegal

substances. However, all have the potential for addiction and all can have a substantial effect on the workplace. In the context of work, the misuse of drugs and alcohol in particular, can not only damage the health of the user, but also have an impact on the workplace in respect of absenteeism and reduced efficiency. Smoking, while certainly not an illegal activity in itself, is, since 2007 (2006 in Scotland), illegal in the workplace. This is covered in more detail later in the chapter.

While there are no firm statistics on the effects of drug misuse in the workplace, there is evidence to show that the misuse of alcohol is associated with increased costs to the business and an increased risk of injury to the individual concerned and his/her colleagues and patients.

- 20–25% of patients in acute hospital beds have alcohol as a contributory factor in their admission.
- 20% of fatal accidents at work involve people with blood alcohol levels over the legal drink drive limit.
- Between 8 and 14 million working days are lost every year because of alcohol-related absenteeism.
- Costs to industry are estimated at over £2 billion per year.
- Smoking costs the National Health Service (NHS) around £1.5 billion per year.

Managing Health and Safety in the Dental Practice: A Practical Guide, by Jane Bonehill   © 2010 by Blackwell Publishing Ltd.

Legislation

- Health and Safety at Work etc. Act 1974:

  Employers have a general duty to their employees, so far as is reasonable, to provide and maintain equipment and systems of work that are safe and without risks to health. The general duty covers the physical and psychological well-being of employees and the individual needs of each employee should be considered.

- Management of Health and Safety at Work Regulations 1999:

  Employers must undertake suitable and sufficient assessments of risks to the health and safety of employees and implement reasonable controls.

- Misuse of Drugs Act 1971:

  It is an offence under the Misuse of Drugs Act 1971 for any person to "knowingly permit the production, supply or use of controlled substances on their premises except in specified circumstances (e.g. when they have been prescribed by a doctor)." (Source: HSE.)

- The Health Act 2006:

  Employers have a legal responsibility to ensure premises are smoke free, and they are accountable for staff and customers.

- The Smoke-free (Premises and Enforcement) Regulations 2006:

  From 1 July 2007 it is an offence to smoke in virtually all 'enclosed' and 'substantially enclosed' workplaces. The terms are defined in the Regulations.

- The Smoke-free (Signs) Regulations 2007 – (self-explanatory):

  Specific smoke-free regulations covering premises, vehicles and signage which were enacted on different dates in 2006 and 2007 in England, Wales, Scotland and Northern Ireland.

Principles of working safely

Apart from the general duties of employers covered in the legislation above, the Health and Safety Executive (HSE) says that 'if you knowingly allow an employee under the influence of excess alcohol to continue working and this places the employee or others at risk, you could be prosecuted'. Clearly, the same could be said for allowing an employee to work under the influence of drugs. A dental surgery is potentially a dangerous environment as it contains many items, which, if not used correctly, could injure the user, his/her colleagues or the patient. Misuse of alcohol or drugs means that the judgement of the individual is affected and it becomes more likely that accidents will happen. Apart from the misuse of equipment such as X-ray machines, needles, drills and so on, there is also potential for these items not to be correctly sterilised. There is further information below about the effects that misuse of alcohol, drugs and smoking can have on a business and on an individual. As dentistry is one of the medical professions, it could also be considered to be a stronger reason for misuse to be dealt with, and to be seen to be dealt with, promptly. The main aims of the General Dental Council (GDC) are listed as follows:

- Protect patients.
- Promote confidence in dental professionals.
- Be at the forefront of health-care regulation.

It should be noted that the protection of patients is the first and most important aim listed.

The effects of alcohol, drugs and smoking

As has been seen above, the misuse of alcohol and drugs can have a significant effect on the behaviour of an individual as well as on his/her health and well-being. However, smoking will also affect the health and well-being of a person, particularly if he/she has been smoking for some time. All three can also have an impact on colleagues and on patients. All three types of substances could be said to be taken for their narcotic or stimulant effect and can lead to addiction if misused.

Alcohol abuse

Many people regard alcohol as a positive and pleasurable part of their lives. It is only when alcohol is abused that it will impact on an individual's behaviour and on his/her ability to work safely. While there are no known figures on the number of workplace accidents where alcohol consumption is a factor, alcohol is known to affect both judgement and physical coordination. The figures in the introduction to this chapter show how costly alcohol abuse can be in the workplace and the effects on the individual are not only quantifiable in terms of money.

It may be difficult for employers to be sure when they spot the signs of alcohol abuse and when observed it can also be a daunting prospect to deal with the situation. Some of the indications might be

- decreased productivity;
- higher rates of absenteeism;
- being late for work regularly;
- increased aggression;
- bad decision-making.

Some physical signs might be

- slurred speech, increased clumsiness or unsteadiness;
- blackouts;
- weight loss (those dependent often drink rather then eat);
- redness in face;
- complaining of tingling in hands and feet.

Observable 'mental' signs might be

- increased irrationality, agitation or anger;
- excessive weeping or emotional display;
- unexplained absences during the day.

Of course, the above signs and symptoms could be an indication of a number of illnesses; so care is needed when confronting someone with the employer's concerns.

Contrary to the popular view that someone who abuses alcohol is out of work and possibly homeless, many such people are employed and so create issues for themselves, their colleagues and their employers. If the person concerned has direct contact with patients, the situation can become very serious indeed for the safety of the patient and the reputation of that dental practice, and ultimately for the profession.

Drug abuse

There are no figures available to show how much absenteeism or how many accidents in the workplace have occurred as a result of the misuse of drugs. However, the implications of drug misuse are wide ranging and will have a significant effect on the individual's physical and mental well-being and on his/her colleagues and their patients. It can cost an employer through increased absenteeism and reduced productivity and increase the risk of accidents. As judgement is affected, there is a potential danger to the well-being of patients, which, of course, cannot be allowed to happen. Drug abuse refers to the use of controlled substances (as described in the Misuse of Drugs Act 1971) and to intentional misuse of prescribed or over-the-counter drugs. It can also apply to the misuse of solvents. Misuse of any of these drugs will impair performance.

The signs and symptoms that may indicate that an individual has a drug problem are variable, but many will be similar to those listed earlier in relation to alcohol abuse. For example,

- decreased productivity.
- higher rate of absenteeism.
- being late for work.
- impaired judgement.
- unexplained weight loss.
- general malaise.
- irrationality and edginess.

As mentioned above, some of these symptoms could be indicative of other illnesses, so it will be important for an employer to look at the whole picture for an individual.

Smoking

The Health Act 2006 brought in statutory rules about smoking in the workplace from 1 July 2007 in England. Similar legislation was brought in from 12 April 2007 in Wales, 26 March 2006 in Scotland and 30 April 2007 in Northern Ireland. There is more on these regulations in the section 'The smoke-free workplace'. However, although smoking is legal outside an enclosed workplace, employers will want to consider how they will manage the situation with employees who are smokers. This may be of particular concern with those employees who, in a dental environment, are in contact with members of the public. Within a dental surgery colleagues work closely together and their proximity to patients can be very high when treating them. Smokers cannot avoid the smell of tobacco lingering on their clothes and on their breath and some patients will find this very unpleasant. It may be better to ask staff not to smoke during working hours.

The consequences of smoking are well known and include diseases of the lungs such as emphysema, bronchitis and lung cancer. Nicotine causes fat deposits to narrow and block the blood vessels and this can lead to heart attacks and strokes. Nicotine is a very addictive drug, which is, of course, why smokers can find it very hard to give up. Many who try to give up initially feel cravings and other withdrawal symptoms. Nicotine affects the chemicals in the brain and this may be why many feel that smoking helps relieve symptoms such as stress.

Some employers provide support for those who wish to stop smoking, by encouraging self-help groups, providing information on sources of help and so on. Smoking cessation sessions are a service offered by many dental practices to patients. These could also be available for members of staff. There are also many other aids available, such as books, counselling, doctors, hypnosis and nicotine substitutes of various kinds.

The smoke-free workplace

Legislation, as shown at the start of this chapter, was introduced in 2007 (2006 in Scotland) in all parts of the United Kingdom with respect to smoking in public places. The rules apply to all enclosed and 'substantially enclosed' places and workplaces, including closed parts of vehicles. Under this legislation, it is an offence to smoke in any of these places, or to **allow** smoking in any of these places or to fail to display a 'no smoking' sign in the way the legislation specifies. The rules apply to smoking any substance, not just tobacco.

Before the legislation changes, some dental practices permitted smoking in staff rest rooms or in a designated smoking room, but this is no longer allowable. If someone wishes to smoke at work he/she would have to go outside the building, although it is not specified as to how far away from the building he/she needs to be. While some employers have provided a shelter outside their buildings, this is something which most health-care professionals may want to avoid, particularly, if it were to be in view of patients arriving for their appointments. Any shelter which is provided must not in itself be 'substantially enclosed.'

Mobile workers will need to be aware of the rules which apply to smoking in vehicles. It is an offence for an employee to smoke in a company vehicle if

- he/she is accompanied by a colleague; or
- if the vehicle is used by more than one employee, even if all those who use the vehicle are smokers.

The rules for smoking in vehicles are quite complicated as they apply to a number of different kinds of vehicle, but the two points above are those most likely to apply in a dental context. No smoking signs must also be displayed in company vehicles. The exact specifications for these vary among the countries in the United Kingdom.

Overall, given the known dangers of smoking and the fact that a dental surgery is a medical environment, a practice may decide to ban smoking at work altogether. For there to be no ambiguity about this, it should be part of a contract of employment. Even if a member of staff smokes outside, the smoke will linger on his/her breath and on the clothes and will be noticeable to colleagues and patients on his/her return inside the building. Professional standards in dealing with patients will mean that this is not acceptable.

Managing alcohol and drug abuse

The author of this handbook has been asked on a number of occasions for advice on how to handle employees who come to work clearly under the influence of something which is affecting their behaviour and their ability to function effectively. This is a sensitive area but one which must be tackled, given that the safety of patients and employees is so important. Mention was made earlier of the importance of a clear policy on misuse of drugs and alcohol. Managing someone who has problems in this area is going to be easier for an employer if a policy exists in which employees have signed to confirm their agreement. Under the Health and Safety at Work etc. Act 1974 there is a general duty placed upon an employer to ensure, as far as is reasonable, the health safety and welfare of the employees. An employer could be prosecuted if he/she knowingly allows an employee, who is under the influence of alcohol or drugs, to continue working if this places the employee or others at risk. There is also a requirement placed upon employees to take reasonable care of themselves and any others who could be affected by their behaviour. Managing this issue, therefore, has a number of aspects:

- Duty of care to employees who may be 'under the influence'
- Duty of care to all other employees who could be affected
- Duty of care to patients – of primary concern to the dental profession

It can be seen therefore that even if someone is not directly concerned with meeting or treating patients, there are still risks in allowing him/her to remain at work if he/she is affected by drugs or alcohol. Someone attending work in the morning with alcohol on his/her breath, for example, may not have been drinking that morning, but may have consumed substantial quantities the night before. Alcohol can remain in the bloodstream for many hours and no amount of black coffee, fresh air or any other apparent 'remedy' can remove it. It is therefore quite possible for someone who

has drunk a lot of alcohol the night before to be unfit for work the next morning. While it would be impossible (and no employer would wish to do this) to regulate an individual's private life, any policy needs to make clear that everyone has a responsibility to arrive at work (or return from lunch) in a state where they are fit to work safely.

Dealing with those who abuse substances of any kind is something which needs to be handled sensitively. While it may be necessary to send someone home for a day if he/she is not able to function safely, consideration needs to be given to whether this is a one-off situation or typical of the behaviour of that individual over a period of time. Addiction to alcohol and drugs is a health issue and needs to be given the same consideration and confidentiality as any other health issue. A good employer will provide support to an employee undergoing treatment for an illness and this support should extend to treatment for addiction. It is unlikely that an employment tribunal or a court would uphold a situation where someone was dismissed unless the employer could show that they had first tried to support their employee to obtain treatment *(Source: HSE)*.

An employer will need to ask himself/herself the following:

- Is this a one-off issue or part of an ongoing problem?
- Can I consult someone else for advice and support?
- What does the policy say about drugs and alcohol?
- Can I provide support or has the situation gone beyond that point?
- Should further discussion be held/further training given to all staff?
- Do I need to consider bringing in 'experts' for the training/discussions?

Screening

Some organisations, particularly in the United States, have introduced screening for drugs and alcohol, either periodically for all employees or for sections of employees, or when recruiting new staff. In this country, there is no legal obligation for employees to agree to screening; employers can only ask employees to undergo this. As an individual who abuses alcohol or drugs is unlikely to agree to screening, this is probably not something most dental practices would want to consider. However, some companies where safety is a significant issue are using screening and testing. Separate consent would need to be obtained for both drugs and alcohol screening. If an organisation does decide to go down this route, they would need to ensure confidentiality of the results and, before embarking on such action, would need to decide what they will do if the screening shows positive results.

Policy

In view of the potentially substantial impact on a business an employer needs to consider drawing up a policy on the use of drugs, alcohol and tobacco which will be clearly understood by all staff (Figure 2.1). While this may seem to be a very formal thing to do, especially for a small practice, it has the advantage that everyone knows the standards of behaviour expected of them. Consideration should be given to implementing this policy even if there are currently no such problems. The time to draw up the policy is not when there is a problem to be dealt with. In order for all staff to be fully committed to the policy, it is good practice to involve them in drawing it up. The HSE booklet *Don't Mix It: A Guide for Employers on Alcohol at Work* contains very simple, straightforward suggestions for drawing up a model alcohol policy, which could be adapted to also apply to misuse of drugs.

In summary, the existence of a policy, which clearly sets out the expectations of all staff, will make managing alcohol and drug-related problems much easier. Figure 2.1 gives some good advice on how to draw up the policy. Employers should support staff to help them overcome any ongoing problems of addiction as far as is practicable, but may have to consider dismissal as a last resort in order to protect other employees and patients.

Professional implications of alcohol and drug abuse

All dentists and dental care professionals must be registered by the GDC in order to practice. Dental care professionals include clinical dental technicians, dental nurses, dental hygienists, dental technicians, dental therapists and orthodontic therapists. The GDC publishes a booklet *Standards for Dental Professionals* and all registrants are expected to follow the principles set out in those standards. This applies irrespective of whether the registrant routinely treats patients or not. Among its aims, the GDC sets out the following:

- 'We aim to protect patients'
- 'We set standards of dental practice' and (among others)
- 'We work to strengthen patient protection'

It also sets out, in the standards document, 'if you believe that patients might be at risk because of your health, behaviour or professional performance, or that of a colleague, or because of any aspect of the clinical environment, you should take action.'

It can be seen that there is a responsibility on all those registered with the GDC to follow its guidelines in order to maintain registration and in order to be allowed to practice. The council does have powers under the 1984 Dentists Act (as amended) to take action when it is alleged that a dental professional's 'fitness to practice' is impaired by reason of his/her professional performance. The GDC gives a list of aspects that could be said to constitute impairment of a registrant's fitness to practice. These include

- misconduct;
- deficient professional performance;
- adverse physical or mental health.

Where this kind of allegation is made the council will have to investigate further and the person complained about may have to undergo a full assessment of his/her performance. From everything that has been said earlier in this chapter,

Figure 2.1   Model alcohol and drugs policy.

The information below is designed to assist the dental practice in developing a policy that meets the needs of the organisation. It has been adapted from the HSE's model alcohol policy. The main headings act as guidance for you to state your specific arrangements.

Aims

Why have a policy? (State your intention and commitment) Who does the policy apply to? (Note: best practice would be for the policy to apply equally to all staff and their respective roles.)

Responsibility

Who is responsible for implementing the policy? (Note: The employer will have overall responsibility but the practice managers will be responsible in some way)

The rules

How does the company expect employees to behave to ensure that their alcohol or drug consumption does not have a detrimental effect on their work?

Special circumstances

Do the rules apply in all situations or are there exceptions?

Confidentiality

A statement assuring employees that any alcohol or drug problem will be treated in strict confidence.

Help

A description of the support available to employees who have problems because of their drinking or drug habit.

Information

A commitment to providing employees with general information about the effects of alcohol and drugs on health and safety.

Disciplinary action

The circumstances in which disciplinary action will be taken.

---

it is clear that abuse of drugs or alcohol could be the cause of any of the above impairments. By abusing alcohol or drugs a dental professional puts himself/herself at risk of suspension or erasure from the Register. If this happens he/she would be unable to practice further in dentistry.

Summary

It is clear therefore that issues around the abuse of drugs and alcohol cannot be taken lightly. With the assistance of a clear workplace policy on the matter and adherence to the guidelines of the GDC, this difficult subject can be more effectively dealt with in the workplace.

Action – check the following

- Do you have a written policy on the abuse of alcohol and drugs, which everyone in your practice has signed up to?
- Do you have a no smoking policy in place?
- Do you have 'no smoking' signs in place, which meet the requirements of the law?

Frequently asked questions

Q. We are only a small practice and I do not know where to go for further advice about a colleague who may be abusing alcohol?

A. Firstly, you need to address the issue with your colleague. Often recognition of the problem and having someone to talk to is part of coming to terms with it and can aid recovery. If this does not produce any change in behaviour then it is advisable to contact your dental defence organisation who will provide expert advice on how to manage the situation. As a last resort, if you are unable to resolve the situation, you can contact the GDC to raise a concern if you believe that patients might be at risk.

Q. Where can I get further advice about drugs and alcohol abuse in the workplace?

A. The HSE produces booklets on both subjects which are available to download from their website.

Q. What should I do if I suspect that a patient who has attended for treatment is under the influence of drugs or alcohol?

A. It may be wise to suggest to the patient that he/she returns on another occasion as his/her behaviour on this occasion may be irrational. It may be that fear of going to the dentist has contributed to the drinking, in which case further discussion may be necessary.

Links to other chapters

Chapter 12 – Managing health and safety
Chapter 15 – Occupational health and well-being
Chapter 17 – Policy
Chapter 20 – Stress management

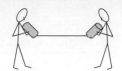

3 Communication and training

Scope of this chapter

- Introduction
- Legislation
- Information, instruction, training and supervision
- Communication process
- Training process

Figures

Introduction

Communicating on health and safety issues is vital for all dental environments regardless of the size of the organisation or the number of people employed. Communication throughout all levels demonstrates a commitment from employers and management in developing policies to achieve a positive health and safety culture. The communication process should enable all members of the team to consult on safe working practices. It helps identify areas where they may need training in order to achieve competence and take an active role in the assessment and control of risks. Effective communication is achieved by a clear, straightforward and unambiguous transfer of information which allows for feedback and involvement of all internal and external parties.

Legislation

Please note that this is not an exhaustive list; there are a range of regulations which contain a requirement for training to be provided and/or competence to be demonstrated. Listed below are a selection of legal requirements.

- Health and Safety at Work etc. Act 1974:

  Employers have a general duty to provide such information, instruction, training and supervision as is necessary to ensure, so far as is reasonable, the health and safety at work of employees.

- Safety Representatives and Safety Committees Regulations 1977:

  If an employer recognises trade unions, the union will appoint a safety representative who will consult with the employer on matters affecting employees. If at least two safety representatives request in writing that a safety committee be formed, the employer must establish the committee within three months of the request.

- The Health and Safety (Consultation with employees) Regulations 1996:

  Where employees are not represented by safety representatives under The Safety Representative and Safety Committees Regulations 1977, the employer is required to consult with employees on matters relating to their health and safety at work.

- The Information and Consultation of Employees Regulations 2004:

  Requires employers of larger organisations, where more than 50 people are employed, to make or amend arrangements to inform and consult the workforce on issues which affect them.

- The Health and Safety Information for Employees (Amendment) Regulations 2009:

  Employers are required to ensure that each employee has easy access to the approved poster or leaflet, telling them what they need to know about health and safety, and how they can obtain the name and address of the 'local' enforcing authority and the address of employment medical advisory service (EMAS). The 1989 existing unrevised poster can be displayed (providing the information is kept up to date) for up to 5 years (until 2014).

- Employers' Liability (Compulsory Insurance) Regulations 1998:

  Employers must make available their certificate of liability insurance at their place of business. It can either be displayed in a prominent place or stored electronically providing it can be retrieved and made available to those who may request to see it.

- Management of Health and Safety at Work Regulations 1999:

  Employers are required to make a suitable and sufficient assessment of the risks to which employees are exposed to help determine the extent of health and safety training to be provided.

- Personal Protective Equipment at Work Regulations 1992 (as amended 2002):

  Employers are required to ensure that employees are provided with adequate information, instruction and training so they can make effective use of the PPE in order to protect them against workplace hazards.

- Health and Safety (Display Screen Equipment) Regulations 1992 (as amended 2002):

  Where a person is a 'user' employers are required to provide adequate health and safety training in the use of the workstation.

- Manual Handling Operations Regulations 1992 (as amended 2002):

  Employers should provide specific information and training as is necessary to ensure that manual handling tasks are carried out safely therefore reducing the risk of injury.

- Control of Substances Hazardous to Health Regulations 2002:

  Where employees may be exposed to hazardous substances the employer must provide information, instruction and training on the risk to health and precautions that must be taken/implemented.

- Ionising Radiations Regulations 1999:

  Employers are required to provide information, instruction and training to all employees involved in the work with ionising radiation, this applies to all people who may be affected. Information, instruction and training should include the risks to health and the precautions that must be taken.

- The Health and Safety (Training for Employment) Regulations 1990:

  Anyone receiving relevant training (work experience provided as part of a training course or programme, or training for employment or both) should be treated as employees for the purposes of health and safety legislation (source: Health and Safety Executive).

Information, instruction, training and supervision

All of these play a part in communicating health and safety and each serves a distinct purpose. However, all are aimed at raising awareness, developing knowledge and understanding, assisting in improving safe working practices and facilitating adherence to policies and procedures.

Information:
- Providing factual data to people about health and safety measures

Instruction:
- Telling people what they can and cannot do

Training:
- Helping people to learn and acquire skills to carry out a particular task

Supervision:
- Ensuring the protection of individuals by providing direction, advice, support and guidance

Information, instruction, training and supervision should be embedded into your day-to-day activities through a planned and structured communication process.

Communication process

The communication process should be an integral part of your health and safety management system. It should include both internal and external people and is relevant when recruiting and selecting staff and when contracting external parties. This helps to demonstrate your commitment to the health, safety, welfare and well-being of all persons on whom your business depends. External parties may be your patients, visitors to the practice or those who you have formed a working contract with. You must ensure that all persons are suitably, appropriately and

effectively informed about any health and safety issues that may affect them (specific issues relating to visitors, locums and contractors are covered in Chapter 21).

Methods of communicating health and safety

An effective method of communicating health and safety is vital to the relationships between employer and employee and anyone else who might be affected. Effective communication helps to manage attitudes and behaviour. In Chapter 17 we have identified how the health and safety policy can be communicated; here, we will cover other means of communication.

- Health and safety promotion campaigns – periodic, routine events addressing topical issues. The use of display boards in public areas, for example, in a waiting room, is a useful resource to highlight the key points and attract interest.
- Practice meetings – a planned process where every member of the team actively contributes. Individuals in turn could be given a specific topic (as set out and arranged for in Part 3 of your policy) to explore and reflect on and provide any updates. Meetings should be held at least monthly with an agenda that clearly reflects the needs of the practice.
- Employee representatives/champions – it may be appropriate or legally required to elect a health and safety representative. This person must be provided with suitable resources in order to carry out his/her duties competently and effectively.
- Posters, signs and notices – appropriately sighted, informing and raising awareness of health and safety issues or instructing people on what they must or must not do. Certain posters and notices are legally required to be displayed or made available for people to view, for example, the Health and Safety Law – *what you need to know* poster and the Employers Liability Insurance Certificate.
- Practice newsletter – addressing any updates to legislation and working practices, recognising particular achievements and good news stories.

■ Presentations – the use of films and slides is useful to provide a more visual approach. They can be used as part of a training programme or to create discussion at meetings.

A combination of the methods mentioned has proved to be most effective in raising awareness as opposed to just using one method in isolation.

Training process

Health and safety training is required by law. Several legislative requirements which state that a person must be trained to deal with the hazard presented have been listed earlier. In addition, there is a range of other reasons for training your staff in health and safety.

■ Enhance knowledge and develop practical skills enabling individuals to carry out their duties safely in compliance with legislation and professional standards.
■ Create a positive safety culture that influences behaviour and attitude towards job roles.
■ Raise performance standards throughout the profession to ensure the health, safety and welfare of all staff and the protection of patients.
■ Encourage individuals to take an active role in identifying hazard and assessing and controlling risks, thereby preventing accidents.
■ Demonstrate the commitment of staff to the General Dental Council's mandatory requirements for continuing professional development (CPD) in relation to the following:
  □ Medical emergencies
  □ Disinfection and decontamination
  □ Radiography and radiation protection
  For those who work in a clinical environment the following are also recommended:
  □ Legal and ethical issues
  □ Complaints handling
■ Broaden the concept of health and safety and apply it to the key elements of clinical governance and risk management.

Structuring the training process

This should be undertaken using the **five-step** approach as follows:

Step 1 – Identify the need for training (Figure 3.1)
■ Decide if legislative requirements exist, for example, where people are involved in any aspect of ionising radiation.
■ Identify if staff have the necessary skills and knowledge to do their job safely; this may be done on a job role basis, but the needs of an individual must also be considered.
■ Identification of training needs can be undertaken as part of performance reviews or appraisals.
■ Results of workplace inspections or audits may identify the need to provide training in specific areas.
■ Examine accident/ill health/significant event records and look for patterns and trends.
■ Are new equipment or procedures being introduced?
■ Do your risk assessments indicate the need for training as a control measure?

Step 2 – Plan the training programme (Figure 3.2)
■ Determine your priorities, including any legal, professional or mandatory requirements or where people may be at a high level of risk if training is not provided.
■ Agree on the aims and objectives of the training and on how you will measure the outcomes.
■ Decide who will deliver the training; should it be in-house personnel or an external training company?
■ Consider the individual's learning style and determine the most suitable training methods and techniques.
■ Identify what resources will be required, including who will be involved to mentor and to provide support and guidance.
■ Determine a suitable and appropriate training programme that meets the needs of the organisation and the individual.

Your team meetings are a type of training provided they follow the above format.

Figure 3.1　Training needs analysis (TNA).

EMPLOYEE NAME: ....　JOB ROLE/TITLE: ....

DATE OF LAST TNA: ....　DATE OF THIS TNA: ....

PERSON CONDUCTING TNA: ....　POSITION IN ORGANISATION: ....

REASON FOR TNA: (please circle)

Induction　　Role change　　Promotion　　Legal/Professional standards　　Risk assessment review　　Organisation change　　Other (specify)

Record responsibility for health and safety	Current skills Level 1, 2, 3 or 4	Current knowledge Level 1, 2, 3 or 4	Training/learning need identified

Level 1	Level 2	Level 3	Level 4
• No training undertaken • No knowledge of the topics	• Close supervision needed • Basic knowledge of the topics	• Skilled to carry out task with limited supervision • Adequate knowledge of the topics	• Operate without supervision • Detailed knowledge and understanding of the topics

Figure 3.2 Personal training plan (PTP).

EMPLOYEE NAME:.. **JOB ROLE/TITLE:**............................

DATE/PERIOD: .... **MANAGER/PERSON CONDUCTING PTP:**............................

Specific training/ learning need	Purpose/objectives	Content and/or training programme	Training provider	Date/s	Completed (date and signature)

Step 3 – Provide training

- Maximise the training time but do not overload the individual with too much information at any one time.
- Use actual examples and case studies where appropriate.
- Ensure sessions are structured appropriately and allow for ongoing feedback to check understanding.
- Meet with the individual at regular intervals to confirm the relevance of training and to show support.

Step 4 – Evaluate training (Figure 3.3)

- Immediate outcomes of the programme should be determined and the following considered: have the training aims and objectives been met and how effective was the training delivery?
- Successive effectiveness should then be measured – did the individuals pass the test, complete assignments or achieve a grade; has the training improved their knowledge and understanding and is this demonstrated in the way they carry out their job (practical skills) and are they now working as they have been trained?
- Management issues for health and safety should also be considered in your evaluation. For example, have there been any improvements in the performance of the organisation? Have accident/ill health/significant event figures reduced and has the training influenced a team approach to health and safety?
- Is further training needed and if so, what are the specifics?
- When will refresher training be needed?

Step 5 – Record outcome (Figure 3.4)

- All training must be recorded, including both in-house training and that provided by an external company.
- In some cases it is a legal requirement to record training, for example, in ionising radiation regulations, Regulation 14 Guidance 14(a)–(b).
- The record should include the name of the attendees and their job title, details of the course subject and date/s provided, length of the event and whether it is verifiable or non-verifiable. Key

learning outcomes, and how they are applied to the job role, should be noted. There should be reference made to certificates gained and the aims and objectives of the event.

As previously mentioned, communicating health and safety should begin at **recruitment and selection**, then lead into the **training** of internal personnel at **induction**. Communication and training must continue throughout an individual's employment.

Induction training

This is quite simply a means of providing new or return-to-work employees (including those who are self-employed) with all relevant health and safety information, instruction and training. This should be done through a consultative approach.

Purpose of induction

This is an opportunity to integrate staff into the organisation by establishing fundamental aspects of how the organisation operates and what is expected of the staff. It should aim to achieve the following:

- Impart the organisation's mission, values, goals and philosophy on health and safety.
- Inform on policies, procedures and expectations relating to safe working practices.
- Raise awareness of legal duties placed on employer and employee.
- Aid staff retention by making people feel cared for as they can see that health and safety is being managed.
- Help to identify, and therefore, respect and manage the individual attitudes and behaviours that people present with.
- Demonstrate compliance with legislation and professional standards.

People who need induction

This will vary between organisations; however, in general terms all persons should be inducted

Figure 3.3   Training evaluation record (TER).

EMPLOYEE NAME: .... JOB ROLE/TITLE: ....

DATE/PERIOD: .... MANAGER/PERSON CONDUCTING PTP: ....

The purpose of this TER is for you to reflect on the training undertaken and measure the outcomes

Training undertaken	Purpose/objectives	Met Yes No	Additional training required (refer PTP)	Any other comments

Figure 3.4 Continuing professional development journal.

NAME: **JOB ROLE/TITLE:**   **DATES FROM:**   **TO:**

Key: V = Verifiable   NV = Non-verifiable

Value grade: 1 = Maintained current skills and knowledge   2 = Enhanced skills and knowledge   3 = Transferred skills and knowledge to new situation

Topic/event/ activity attended	Date/s	Provider	Hours	V/NV	Value Grade	Key learning outcomes	How applied

whether employed or self-employed. It should include those on a training programme and both full-time and part-time staff. Those responsible for induction should be aware that some individuals may be more vulnerable than others for specific reasons as listed below:

- Part-time staff, because of lack of continuity
- Those new to the profession, who will be unfamiliar with working practices and occupational hazards
- Young persons and Work Experience students, who may be immature and lack knowledge, skills and experience
- Temporary/locum staff, who may be unfamiliar with the practice's specific systems, policies and procedures
- Returnees to work, as changes may have occurred and adapting and adjusting takes time; for some, the transition period is difficult
- Those transferring to other job roles – working with new equipment or having increased responsibilities for others
- Contractors (see Chapter 21)

The induction should take into consideration individual needs and be tailored accordingly to ensure it is appropriate to the specific role.

Structuring the induction

The communication and induction training process consists of three stages described using the abbreviation **P.I.P.**

Pre-employment (recruitment and selection):

- Place your Health and Safety Policy Statement (Part 1) on your website or in your practice leaflet as this will inform applicants and prospective employees of your commitment to health and safety
- Provide an overview of your organisational standards at interview as this will help interviewees to decide if they are prepared to commit to these standards
- Ask competency-based questions at the interview to explore knowledge, attitudes and behaviours towards health and safety.

Once you have selected the successful applicant, in order to demonstrate your commitment carry out the following:

- Send out the offer letter and include the following:
  - □ Parts 1 and 2 of your Health and Safety Policy
  - □ Medical/health questionnaire to ascertain any conditions you need to be aware of in order to reduce risks and care for the individual (**please note that this must not be used as part of the selection process**)
  - □ Induction plan setting out where, when and how the induction will be carried out (Figure 3.5)
- Encourage the new employees to prepare by devising a list of questions they want to ask and deciding who they would like to meet.
- Invite the new employees to attend a session before commencing employment in order to familiarise themselves with the environment and meet the team.
- Appoint a competent 'buddy' (colleague) to provide support and guidance.
- Circulate the induction plan to those who will be involved in the training in order to gain commitment and cooperation.

Initial employment (probation period):

- Determine an appropriate probation period in line with the contract of employment; for example, this might be 3 months.
- Commence the induction on day 1 of the person's starting employment.
- Emphasise roles and responsibilities and organisational commitment to health and safety in line with Parts 1 and 2 of the Health and Safety Policy.
- Introduce mandatory health and safety essentials in line with the induction plan as described in 'elements of an induction' (**R.O.M.E.**).
- Allow the inductee to shadow other employees.
- Meet back with the buddy and manager at intervals throughout the period to seek clarification, discuss any problems and confirm understanding.
- Incorporate all three learning styles (show, tell and do) in the delivery of the induction.

- Ensure your induction is a consistent and continuous process throughout the probation period as this avoids overloading the new member of staff with too much information at any one time.

Post probation (end of probation period):

- Evaluate the effectiveness of the induction training.
- Carry out post-induction reviews to gain feedback and measure the individual's performance.
- Identify and analyse further health and safety training needs (Figure 3.1).
- Determine whether the aims and objectives of the induction have been achieved; if not establish the reasons.

Health and safety induction should begin as soon as possible after the person has started his/her employment. The actual length of time for the induction will be determined by the individual organisation and this may be aligned to their probationary period. However, regardless of the time period there should be a framework in place, which consists of essential **elements** that can be carried out with all individuals and which are flexible to meet specific needs.

Elements of an induction

Your health and safety induction programme should have clearly defined and well thought out aims and objectives. This not only enables you to measure the effectiveness but also provides evidence of verifiable CPD for the individual/s concerned. The essential elements are contained in **R.O.M.E** as follows:

Roles and responsibilities (who does what):

- Who's who in your organisation (organisation structure)
- Responsibilities for general and specific health and safety functions (Part 2 of your Health and Safety Policy)
- Lines of reporting and contact details
- Sources of advice and information, both internal and external

- The inductee's role, responsibility and legal duties for health and safety
- Identification of training needs specific to the inductee's role

Organisation commitment (aim is to protect and care for people):

- Mission, values, principles and vision (Part 1 of your Health and Safety Policy)
- Tangible demonstration of commitment (show how it is being applied)
- Health and safety development plan
- Communication and consultation methods
- Health and safety management systems and procedures
- Acceptable working practices

Mandatory health and safety essentials (what must be covered):

- Legal and professional standards
- Health and safety policies and procedures (Part 3 of your Health and Safety Policy)
- Essentials which must be covered during first day and first week of employment

Evaluation of training (determines effectiveness).

- Should verify if objectives are being met
- Should be introduced early in the induction period
- Should be conducted throughout the probationary period
- Should be an ongoing and continuous process (determined by period of induction)
- Should include final confirmation of understanding and agreement (Figure 3.5)

It should be recognised that some individuals may not need such close support as others; therefore, the induction plan can be adapted to meet individual needs (Figure 3.5).

Ongoing training

A periodic review of training needs (Figure 3.1) must be incorporated into your management system. This will ensure that training remains

Figure 3.5   Induction plan and confirmation record.

This document should be used for all new personnel as described in 'People who need inducting' and adapted to ensure it is fit for purpose for both the new recruit and the organisation.

The whole team should be included throughout the induction period and encouraged to provide support where appropriate.

Each item should be signed and dated by the person with responsibility.

For the items/objectives which are not covered comments should be made giving reasons and a date for completion.

The completed confirmation record should be signed by the inductee, practice manager and buddy and a copy kept in the personnel file.

NAME OF INDUCTEE:	JOB TITLE:		START DATE:	
NAME OF PRACTICE MANAGER:		NAME OF BUDDY AND OTHERS INVOLVED:		
Pre-employment (before starting)				
AIM/ITEM	**OBJECTIVE/DETAILS**		**RESPONSIBILITY**	**COMPLETED** (initial and date or comments)
1.1 Preparation for employment	• Send Parts 1 and 2 of policy, organisation chart, job description and induction plan • Encourage new recruit to analyse information and prepare questions		Practice manager and employer	
1.2 Identify and assess individual medical health needs	• Send medical health questionnaire to be returned at familiarisation session on Day 1		Practice manager and employer	
1.3 Provide support and guidance	• Determine suitable and appropriate 'buddy' • Brief the team on new recruit • Circulate induction plan to relevant people		Practice manager and employer	
1.4 Familiarise with organisation	• Invite new recruit to attend session prior to starting • Introduce to key staff members and conduct 'general' walk tour		Practice manager and employer	

First day (initial employment)

AIM/ITEM	OBJECTIVE/DETAILS	RESPONSIBILITY	COMPLETED (Initial and date or comments)
2.1 Welcome and introductions	• Meet with employer and practice manager and emphasise commitment to health and safety • Respond to prepared questions and confirm understanding of responses • Check medical health pre-existing conditions and act accordingly • Introduce to buddy and explain role • Introduce to all other staff	Practice manager and employer	

2.2 Familiarise with environment, safety, security and welfare facilities and procedures	• Walk tour in practice to point out following locations and procedures:
	  o Washing, toilet, changing facilities
	  o Eating and rest areas
	  o Entrances, exits, fire escape routes and assembly points
	  o Fire action notices and fire extinguishers
	  o First aid kit, appointed person and accident book
	  o Emergency drug store
	  o Spillage kits
	  o Compressor/plant room
	  o Isolating switches, electricity, water, gas
	  o Start up, close down and locking up
	  o Radiation controlled zones
	  o Personal security measures
	  o Alarm system
	  o PPE/C store
	  o Waste segregation and storage
	  o Occupation health (if provided)
	  o Prohibitions/restricted areas
	  o Clinical and non-clinical work areas
		Buddy	

2.3 Inform of working times	• Discuss and agree on start, finish breaks and lunch times	Practice manager	
2.4 Communicate risk assessments	• Discuss risk assessments in relation to job role and review individual/personal needs	Buddy	
2.5 Observe safe working procedures	• Work shadow buddy to familiarise with organisation requirements	Buddy	

(continued overleaf)

Figure 3.5   (*continued*)

First week (initial employment)

AIM/ITEM	OBJECTIVE/DETAIL	RESPONSIBILITY	COMPLETED (Initial and date or comments)
3.1 Identify training needs	• Conduct training needs analysis on day 2 to identify specific safety training as identified through risk assessments • Devise personal training plan • Provide in-house training throughout the week using all three learning methods	Practice manager Practice manager and buddy	
3.2 Communicate policy arrangements, Part 3 of policy (throughout the week)	• Inform on policy statements and procedures • New recruit to apply safe working procedures while being work shadowed	Practice manager and buddy	
3.3 Consolidation, understanding, confirmation and agreement	• Set time aside throughout the week for discussion and clarification • At end of week verify all subjects have been explained and fully understood • Seek confirmation of acceptance to organisation policy and demonstrate the organisation commitment	Practice manager and buddy Practice manager Practice manager and employer	

Rest of probationary period (initial employment)

3.4 Consistent and continuous induction process	• Continuation of 3.1, 3.2 and 3.3 throughout the induction period	As above	
3.5 Review individual training needs	• Refer to initial training needs analysis and evaluate training already provided • Identify further training needs to ensure new recruits safety • Devise continuing personal training plan	Practice manager and buddy Practice manager Practice manager	

Post-probation period (end of probation)

4.1 Evaluate effectiveness of induction	• Encourage feedback from the new recruit on the overall success of the induction, identify if aims and objectives have been met and determine improvements	Practice manager, employer and buddy
	• Meet with rest of team to disseminate information	Practice manager

Additional comments

(Please record all relevant information i.e. feedback from the inductee on the outcome of the induction)

Declaration

I/We certify that the above health and safety induction has been carried out and all items have been explained in full.

Practice manager signature: Buddy signature:

Date: Date:

I confirm my understanding and acceptance of all policies and procedures covered in the induction and agree to adhere to safe working practices.

Inductee signature: Date:

relevant to the needs of the individual and the organisation. Ongoing training may also be required for the following reasons:

- If a person changes job role, for example, transfers from one department to another
- Promotion – therefore has increased responsibilities and accountabilities
- Specialised training for certain personnel, that is, dental nurse radiographer
- Refresher training to ensure that knowledge and skills are up to date and valid (CPD)
- As previously stated in the section 'Structuring the training process' Step 1

Summary

The Health and Safety Policy of your practice/organisation should clearly state how you communicate with internal and external people on health and safety and how you train your team. Methods used should be relevant and appropriate to the needs of the organisation and individuals concerned. Communication and training should help you to develop standards and improve performance and motivate people to take responsibility and work as a team.

Action – check the following

- Does your Health and Safety Policy include a policy arrangement for communication and training?
- Do you communicate health and safety effectively and are your messages clear, unambiguous and understood?
- Is your induction process suitable and sufficient?
- Do you adopt a structured approach for the ongoing training of your staff?

Frequently asked questions

Q. Should we use an external training company in preference to our in-house staff?

A. It will depend on the particular training need identified. If the expertise exists within your team then on-the-job training can be given. However, if the need is beyond the competence of your staff then it may be necessary to enlist the services of an external trainer.

Q. How do we determine appropriate training methods and techniques and how do we know these are suitable for individuals?

A. It is generally considered that people predominantly learn in three different ways; visual by seeing something, auditory by hearing something and kinaesthetic by doing something. Individuals will favour a particular style; however, a combination of all three is generally preferable when delivering health and safety training. This not only adds interest to a seemingly 'dry' subject but also helps to reinforce messages and aids retention of information.

Q. Are dental practices legally required to establish a health and safety committee and appoint a safety representative?

A. No. Safety committees are usually established in larger organisations where it is seen to be the most appropriate and effective method of consulting with the workforce. Where employees are recognised by a trade union they will be represented by a union safety representative. In non-union workplaces there must be a way of consulting with employees on health and safety. This may take place directly with employees or through an elected representative. Whichever method is selected, you must ensure that a process is in place that allows employers to consult with employees. If a safety representative is elected his/her role must be clearly defined, appropriate resources provided and he/she should be competent to carry out the role.

Links to other chapters

Chapter 12 – Managing health and safety
Chapter 17 – Policy
Chapter 19 – Risk assessment
Chapter 21 – Visitors, locums and contractors

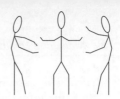

4 Conflict management

Scope of this chapter

- Introduction
- Legislation
- Definitions
- Causes and effects
- Managing conflict

Figures

Figure 4.1 – Conflict risk assessment and action plan.

Introduction

Work-related aggression and violence is a major issue in most sectors, with the highest assault levels being experienced in the health-care sector. Evidence shows that incidents have increased over recent years to an unacceptably high level. The estimated number of incidents of violence experienced by people at work in England and Wales was 655,000 in 2004–2005 (*Source: British Crime Survey (BCS) 27 October 2005*). The dental teams deal directly with service users, for example, customers and patients in their everyday working lives, and are therefore likely to face the risk of verbal and physical ill treatment. The Health and Safety Executive (HSE) is committed to raising awareness of work-related violence and supports a number of initiatives to reduce the level of incidents relating to conflict. A conflict situation can take minutes to escalate from a misunderstanding to aggression and violence. Employers have a duty of care to identify situations that may exist and look at ways of addressing them in order to significantly reduce the incidence of verbal and physical abuse.

Legislation

- Health and Safety at Work etc. Act 1974:

  Employers have a general duty to ensure, so far as is reasonably possible, the health, safety and welfare of all employees. The general duty covers and includes protecting employees from violent behaviour whilst at work.

- Management of Health and Safety at Work Regulations 1999:

  Employers [are] to make suitable and sufficient assessments of risks to the health and safety of employees to identify the measures needed to remove the risks or reduce to an acceptable level. The assessment should, where foreseeable, include the need to protect employees from exposure to violence and aggression.

- Reporting of Injuries, Diseases and Dangerous Occurrences Regulations 1995 (RIDDOR):

  Employers are required to report certain specified accidents and dangerous occurrences to the enforcing authority, via the HSE's incident contact centre, if they arise out of or in connection with work activities this includes acts of physical violence.

- The Corporate Manslaughter (England, Wales and Northern Ireland) and Corporate Homicide (Scotland) Act 2007:

  The organisation must manage or organise their activities in order to prevent serious accidents which could result in death of an employee, and will be guilty of an offence if a person's death amounts to a gross breach of a relevant duty of care owed by the organisation (employer) to the deceased.

Definitions

The dental teams are exposed to situations of conflict everyday of their working lives; however, it is often not realised until it escalates into a more serious situation. Have you ever been faced with an unsatisfied patient? It may have started as a minor disagreement; for example, what he/she expected was not what he/she received. Did you feel intimidated by the abusive words, tone of voice and were you threatened by physical gestures like finger wagging? If so, you may be a victim of workplace violence. The HSE defines workplace violence as 'Any incident in which a person is abused, threatened or assaulted in circumstances relating to their work'. You will notice that this definition is quite wide ranging as it includes any form of abusive or threatening behaviour towards a person. The HSE expands the definition by saying what constitutes workplace violence as a situation where a person

- uses abusive language or behaviour towards another;

- makes a threat towards another;
- physically assaults another.

Types of violent behaviour
- Intimidation – physical or verbal threat
- Bullying and exclusion – imposing opinions or 'sent to Coventry'
- Verbal abuse – name calling, shouting, swearing or belittling language
- Physical gestures – raising or shaking fist or pointing finger
- Physical abuse – touching, pushing, prodding, slapping, punching or kicking
- Stalking – unwanted attention, for example, anonymous or owned messages or being followed

Any form of conflicting or violent behaviour should not be tolerated; staff has a right to work safely. To tackle the issue of conflict and violence it is important to recognise how incidents might occur and the effects it can have on individuals and the business.

Causes and effects

In the dental environment, conflict can occur for a variety of reasons, usually due to misunderstandings and disagreements between people. It should be recognised that the cause is not always attributed to patients. The following provide an overview of some of the underlying causes.

Caused by service providers (dental professionals)

- Staff not trained in customer service delivery
- Training needs analysis not undertaken
- Lack of essential customer service skills
- Unable to interpret customer needs and wants
- Waiting times and delay in service not communicated
- Unable to deal with complaints effectively and ethically
- Difficulty balancing regulatory requirements and patients' needs
- Poor communication, for example,

□ Information not actively distributed or communicated
□ Customers inappropriately informed about service delivery
□ Changes to service not communicated
□ Lack of information when there is delay in service delivery
□ Reluctance to apologise for mistakes
□ Inappropriate responses to problems
□ Inconsistencies in information given
□ Preconceived attitudes about people, which is reflected in behaviours

Caused by service users (customers/patients)

■ Preconceived ideas and expectations
■ Unreasonable expectations
■ Overly dependent on the service provider
■ Reluctance to take advice
■ Unwilling to compromise
■ Cultural differences and misunderstandings
■ Arrives late or does not attend
■ Feeling insecure because of being unfamiliar with surroundings, equipment and the environment
■ Lack of knowledge and understanding of treatment procedures
■ Fear of losing control
■ Out of their comfort zone
■ Suffering from pain
■ Drug or alcohol abuse
■ Predisposed conditions, that is, physical and emotional ill health
■ Personal problems
■ Personality traits, for example, arrogant, selfish, rude, prejudiced and temperamental

Caused by disagreements within the dental team

■ Telling someone else about another individual
■ Everyone having their own ideas
■ Viewing things differently
■ Having diverse expectations
■ Reacting to situations in a variety of ways
■ Differences due to age, gender, background, experience, etc.
■ Different priorities
■ Inappropriate management style

There are many factors that can cause a situation of conflict, and in most instances this is not a deliberate intent on behalf of the individuals concerned. It is important for the practice to recognise how it may occur and how to reduce the risk.

Effects of conflict

Conflict is unhelpful, unhealthy and destructive to the business – if conflict is not managed it can have short-, medium- and long-term effects on individuals and the business; the range of effects include

■ low staff morale;
■ lack of concentration and motivation;
■ absenteeism due to fear of repetition;
■ high staff turnover;
■ emotional or physical pain;
■ depression;
■ stress;
■ legal implications;
■ financial implications, for example, costs associated with
　□ investigation following an incident;
　□ recruitment costs for staff replacement if victims leave;
　□ lower productivity which could result in lost profits;
　□ increased insurance premiums if it results in a claim for compensation;
　□ legal fees to defend a litigation claim.

Managing conflict

Health and safety legislation places responsibilities on everyone to manage workplace risks; therefore, the whole dental team has a legal duty to manage conflict. In addition to the legal duties, compliance with the General Dental Council (GDC) Professional Standards is essential in order to fulfil the requirements of statutory registration. The standards state and provide guidance on how service must be provided to patients. You may be asked by the GDC to account for your behaviour and demonstrate that you have practised in line with the above principles if a situation of conflict arises. If you are unable to provide proof, your registration may be at risk. Clinical governance is another quality standard which sets out the level of quality care that all dental professionals are expected to deliver. Clinical governance requires dental providers to ensure that patients receive quality care. The care must be

- safe – risk prevention and/or control;
- equitable – fair and reasonable;
- patient centred – responsive to needs, wants and preferences.

Therefore, conflict must be managed in order to ensure that the requirements of clinical governance are achieved and maintained.

A risk-based approach is necessary in order to identify the extent of the problem and determine how to avoid and defuse situations. It also includes having a mechanism in place to support those who are victims of conflict. Employers have a duty of care to protect their staff from the risk of conflict. If the following steps are taken it will greatly assist with risk reduction and make the workplace a safer place.

Reducing the risk

The risk of conflict can be greatly reduced through three means: policy, risk assessment and training.

Policy

Policy forms the basis of the organisation's approach to managing conflict; it should state the commitment of the employer and the procedures to follow. For the policy to be effective, it must meet the following criteria:

- Should demonstrate intention and commitment to all persons
- Should define the organisation's approach to violence
- Should set out standards of care and service delivery

- Should communicate unacceptable levels of conflict
- Should show how situations are identified and assessed
- Should inform on the arrangements in place to manage situations
- Should express the benefits of managing conflict
- Should state the responsibilities of all persons
- Should provide support for 'victims'
- Should encourage active consultation
- Should be reviewed routinely and revised if necessary

Policy development
In order to ensure that the policy is understood by everyone the following should take place:

- Clearly state that the aim of the policy is to reduce the likelihood of occurrences.
- Provide training for all staff, starting at induction and ongoing.
- Procedures must be clearly defined and reviewed.
- Advertise by actively informing people of your policy and display the statement of intent (promote).
- Communicate by holding meetings to raise awareness and voice concerns.
- Report all types of violent or confrontational incidents and explore causes.
- Provide commitment from management to address and resolve incidents.
- Recognise the benefits to the team and the business.

The policy must be explicit in the fact that it is a supportive two-way process which requires a commitment from everyone including service providers and users and the dental team.

Risk assessment

Chapter 19 provides details of the process of risk assessment; it is therefore advised that you follow this format (Figure 4.1).

Once the policy is in place the next step is to identify situations when staff may be faced

Figure 4.1   Conflict risk assessment and action plan.

Assessor:	Location/Work area:		RA number:
Date of assessment:		**Date of review:**	

Hazard rate (HR)	Risk rate (RR)	Action priority (AP)	Overall risk rating
A Death, major injury and major damage **B** Over 3-day injury; damage to property/equipment **C** Minor injury, minor damage to property	**1.** Extremely likely to occur **2.** Frequent/often/likely to occur **3.** Slight chance of occurring	**A1** – Unacceptable; must receive immediate attention before work continues **A2/B1** – Urgent; must receive attention as soon as possible to remove hazard or reduce risk **A3/C1** – Must receive attention to reduce risk **B2** – Should receive attention to reduce risk **B3/C2** – Low priority; reduce risk after other priorities **C3** – Very low priority;] reduce hazard or risk after other priorities	

Hazards	Risk factors	Persons at risk	HR	RR	AP	Controls in place and is action required? (Y/N)
1. Duties/Tasks						
1.1						
1.2						
1.3						
1.4						
1.5						
1.6						
1.7						
1.8						
1.9						
1.10						

(continued overleaf)

Figure 4.1 *(continued)*

2. Environment						
2.1						
2.2						
2.3						
2.4						
2.5						
2.6						
2.7						
2.8						
2.9						
2.10						
3. Other						
3.1						
3.2						
3.3						
3.4						
3.5						
3.6						
3.7						
3.8						
3.9						
3.10						

Conflict risk assessment action plan

RA number

No	Control required	Target date	Monitoring date	Revised risk rating	Review date

with conflict and to analyse the extent of the problem and determine what can be done to eliminate the threat or reduce the risk. A conflict risk assessment requires the following:

- An understanding of individual roles in order to identify situations when conflict may occur
- A thorough examination of duties and tasks undertaken by all staff
- An examination of the physical environment and layout of areas
- Consideration of all eventualities so far as is possible

Reducing the risk

- Alter work activities and reorganise tasks and working methods.
- Ensure there are adequate number of personnel available at all relevant times.
- Make changes to the physical environment to remove hazardous items or dangerous areas.
- Install protective devices, for example, surveillance cameras, alarms/warning systems and personal protective devices.
- Ensure people have the necessary skills to manage people effectively.
- Review periodically and revise the assessment if anything changes.

Work as a team to constantly develop the conflict management strategy.

Training

Ensure that staff know how to recognise the early signs of behavioural changes that could indicate conflict and deal effectively with situations in order to prevent or resolve. Training must

- analyse specific needs relevant to respective roles and responsibilities;
- be fit for purpose for both the organisation and individuals;
- incorporate the essential elements of customer service delivery;
- cover effective complaints handling and current procedures;
- be constantly reviewed and remain up to date.

Training should address all eventualities that individuals may be faced with and aim to reduce the risk.

Resolving conflict

It is not always possible to prevent conflict from happening – human beings are sometimes unpredictable and therefore some incidents could not have been foreseen in the risk assessment. Therefore, it is important that staff know how to deal with the situation they are faced with. The following, known as the *C.A.L.M.E.R. approach* to conflict resolution, should be applied:

- **C**larify the issues
- **A**ddress the problem
- **L**isten to the other side
- **M**anage your way to solving
- **E**thically resolve
- **R**ecord the incident

The aim of this approach is to defuse and de-escalate the situation by responding appropriately; this is achieved by the following actions:

- Recognise causative factors.
- Maintain self-control and stay calm.
- Show empathy and actively listen.
- Win his/her trust.
- Recognise the other person's point of view.
- Signal non-aggression by managing verbal and non-verbal behaviour.
- Keep an open mind and manage own attitude.
- Resolve amicably, ethically and legally.

In most instances, the above response will resolve the situation and a suitable outcome achieved. If this is not the case and your personal safety is at risk, then a dynamic risk assessment may be needed; this is covered in Chapter 19 and a summary presented below.

Dynamic risk assessment

- It addresses un-eventualities that could not have been foreseen.
- It requires a continuous assessment of the situation as it unfolds.

- The person adjusts responses to meet the risk presented.
- Time is a factor to ensure the safety of the individual; frustration can escalate to violence very quickly.
- Aim is to respond quickly and appropriately.

Dynamic risk assessment requires the following:

- Observe aggressive signals, facial expressions and actions.
- Listen for aggressive words, tone and pitch.
- Maintain distance and establish 'safe' space and do not let the aggressor enter your zone.
- Call for help or assistance.
- Consider the safety of others in the immediate area.
- Determine a safe exit route and use it if necessary.

If you are in any doubt and your safety is threatened, leave the situation; do not attempt to stay and try to resolve it.

Reporting and recording incidents

It is vital that all incidents are reported internally to a competent named person in order to investigate and analyse the causative factors and learn from experiences to prevent recurrence. Incidents must be reported immediately and an accident/incident record completed, which contains the following details:

- Facts about the victim and the aggressor
- A background to the situation
- Information about and a description of behaviour and the level of any force used in self-defence (not recommended, level of force may have to be justified)
- Comprehensive, accurate and factual account of the event as the report may be used in court
- Data protection of record

The incident must be treated and analysed as a significant event and the following must be incorporated.

- Investigate and analyse the causes and involve all parties.
- Track progress of dealing with the incident.
- Set a date for a review of findings.
- Develop an action plan stating timed developments planned for future.
- Review and audit to check if action plan is on track.
- Give feedback to victim and advise on all actions and the support provided.

The Reporting of Injuries Diseases and Dangerous Occurrences Regulations 1995 (RIDDOR) requires employers to report acts of physical violence if they result in death, major injury or a person being off work for more than three consecutive days.

Post-incident support

People react to situations of conflict differently; therefore, the level and type of support will depend on the needs of the victim. However, in all cases you should put in place 'sympathetic' mechanisms to help victims of workplace conflict recover from situations by applying the following:

- Demonstrate interest and show you care.
- Recognise the signs of distress and the effect the incident has had on the person.
- If the person is off work make contact to enquire about his/her well-being.
- An understanding of people's reactions is important when supporting someone through the stages of recovery.
- Offer appropriate mechanisms to meet their specific needs.

Support mechanisms

- Colleagues and line managers or
- Specialists for longer term recovery stages, for example, counselling, psychiatric or psychological services

The post-incident support process described above can be applied to any situation of conflict;

however, it should be tailored to the specific incident and the needs of the practice.

Summary

It is a fact that conflicting and violent behaviour in society is increasing, the increase is changing peoples' values, change in values destroys communities, these communities consist of individuals who could be your customers and, therefore, customers could be bringing violence into the dental practice. By raising awareness of the importance of managing conflict into your organisation, you can significantly reduce incidences of verbal or physical abuse and of absenteeism caused by these stressful situations; therefore, improve the quality of care you provide for your patients.

Action – check the following

- Do you have a conflict management policy that demonstrates your commitment to your staff?
- Have you assessed the risk of conflict to staff in each area of work?
- Have you identified the underlying causes of conflict for staff and service users?
- Have you undertaken a training needs analysis for each role performed in your practice?

Frequently asked questions

Q. What is meant by justifiable self-defence?
A. It is not advisable to use any level of force in a conflict situation unless you have received specialised training on how to administer it correctly – the most appropriate action is to remove yourself from the situation. It is up to the courts to decide if the force used was justifiable. The decision will be based on whether it was reasonable, determined by what a rational person would have done in the circumstances; therefore permissible and needed in the circumstances and finally proportionate to the seriousness of the situation.

Q. We are thinking about installing a close circuit television (CCTV) in the reception area. Is this sufficient to protect staff from conflict?
A. CCTV is classed as a physical protective measure to monitor normal work activities and react if a situation warrants. It can act as a deterrent and therefore reduce the risk of an incident; however, it is insufficient to solely rely on this device to manage conflict. A well-thought-out risk assessment will help you to explore all eventualities and then determine the most suitable controls. CCTV could be one of the controls in order to protect but not necessarily prevent.

Links to other chapters

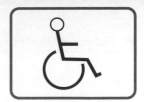

5 Disability access

Introduction

There are approximately 10 million people with disabilities in the United Kingdom; it is estimated that the spending power of these people amounts to £50 billion per year *(Source: Disability Rights Commission, DRC)*. Premises that are accessible to everyone will make the practice more convenient and therefore could put you ahead of your competitors. The risks of doing nothing could result in a claim for compensation, which, according to the Department of Trade and Industry, is reaching an all-time high in successful claims. Employers and dental practice service providers must ensure that they do not directly discriminate by treating an employee, prospective employee or a service user less favourably because of his/her disability. In 2010, the disability discrimination law will be amended to include indirect discrimination.

Legislation

- Health and Safety at Work etc. Act 1974:

  Employers are required to protect the health, safety and welfare of employees and anyone else who may be affected, so far as is reasonably practicable. Any matters affecting an individual are owed the same duty of care as other employees and where necessary employers must take additional measures to protect that employee.

- Disability Discrimination Act 1995 (DDA) (as amended, see below):

  Employers and service providers are required to treat disabled persons fairly in the same way as non-disabled persons and take reasonable steps to remove or alter physical barriers that restrict or prevent access.

☐ *December 1996 – it is unlawful to treat disabled people less favourably for a reason related to their disability*

☐ *October 1999 – make 'reasonable adjustments' to enable disabled people to use your services*

☐ *October 2004 – make 'reasonable adjustments' to the physical features of your premises to overcome barriers to access*

- Workplace (Health, Safety and Welfare) Regulations 1992:

  Employers, owners/occupiers of premises are required to take account of disabled persons and to ensure the workplace is organised in such a way that provides reasonable access.

- Management of Health and Safety at Work Regulations 1999:

  Employers must undertake suitable and sufficient assessments of risks to the health and safety of employees and others who may be affected and determine what measures should be taken to comply with duties under other health and safety legislation.

- The Regulatory Reform (Fire Safety) Order 2005 (RRFSO):

  Employers, occupiers or owners of buildings will need to carry out a fire risk assessment to ensure that people with a disability are able to evacuate the building safely in the event of fire.

Defining disability

A person is disabled if he/she has a physical or **mental impairment** which has a **long-term and substantial adverse effect** on his/her ability to carry out **normal day-to-day activities**. This is further defined as follows:

Impairment:
- Blind and partially sighted
- Deaf and hard of hearing
- Mobility difficulties, including wheelchair users
- Mental health problems

- Severe disfigurements
- Progressive illnesses, for example, human immunodeficiency virus (HIV), multiple sclerosis, cancer and muscular dystrophy[1]
- Long-term health conditions, for example, diabetes
- Learning difficulties
- Loss of memory

Long-term and substantial adverse effects:
- Lasted or likely to last at least 12 months or be recurring
- The rest of a person's life – this may be less than 12 months
- The effect is not trivial or minor

Normal day-to-day activities:
- Carried out by most people frequently; examples are as follows:
  ☐ Going up and down stairs
  ☐ Holding and turning a door handle
  ☐ Using sanitary facilities/WC

Disability is not always obvious; therefore, we cannot assume that a disability does not exist because it is not visible. Take, for example, a 35-year-old female who appears to look fit and healthy but suffers from a chronic lung condition, having contracted an illness as a child. Or an elderly person who, we might assume, is not disabled because the signs are that of the usual ageing process. A person does not have to be registered disabled to be covered by the regulations. Dental practices should therefore take a proactive approach to disability awareness and not wait until someone is unable to access the service.

Discrimination

It is highly unlikely that a dental professional would directly discriminate against a disabled person. However, you may not know if you are discriminating as the law is quite complex; therefore, it is important to have some clarification on what constitutes discrimination. Employers and service providers may be deemed to have

---

[1] Progressive illnesses are covered by the regulations from when the condition is diagnosed.

discriminated in either of two ways *(Source: Disability action)*:

- **Less favourable treatment** – if, for a reason relating to a person's disability, he/she is treated less favourably than others to whom that reason does not apply, and they cannot show that the treatment is justified; and/or
- **Reasonable adjustment** – if they fail to make a 'reasonable adjustment' to the working environment or physical features of premises which place a person with disability at a substantial disadvantage compared to persons without disability, and this failure cannot be justified.

Responsibilities

The DDA places responsibilities on all employers and those providing a service, whether this service is paid for or free. The main purpose of the act is to ensure that individuals with a disability are treated fairly. This is achieved by taking 'reasonable' steps to provide access to your premises. This involves removing or altering physical barriers that restrict or prevent access or consider how you might provide the service in another way. When determining what is reasonable the following general factors should be considered:

- The cost and practicality of making adjustments
- Resources available to accommodate the adjustments
- The effectiveness of changes for disabled people
- Disruption to other service users
- Life of the property and/or business

Specific examples of making reasonable adjustments will be covered in more detail in the following sections.

Employer

The amended legislation in October 2004 meant that organisations employing fewer than 15 employees are no longer exempt form the law. Disabled employees share the same employment

rights as non-disabled people; therefore, it is unlawful to discriminate against them for reasons related to their disability. As a starting point, employers should consider the following health and safety factors in all aspects of the employment process:

- Interview arrangements and access to and around premises
- Work facilities, for example, rest areas and toilets accessible to everyone

Employers should also identify factors that could put the disabled person more at risk by assessing the individual's capabilities, not disabilities, (Figure 5.1) and then, if necessary, undertake a risk assessment to identify at-risk areas and situations, in particular, the following factors:

- The nature of the work, the way it is organised and managed and how this may impact on the employee
- Duration and frequency of tasks and hazardous situations
- The employee's physical, psychological and social well-being and how this affects the ability to carry out his/her role
- The resources, training and any adjustments that can be provided to support the employee

See Chapter 19 for the stages of risk assessment.

- Evacuation procedures in the event of an emergency (also considered below)

If the outcome of the risk assessment shows that more needs to be done to protect the employee from harm, consider making reasonable adjustments to the workplace or the way work is organised.

Reasonable adjustments

An employee with a disability should be encouraged to inform the employer of his/her disability in order for reasonable adjustments to be made. He/she will need to provide as much information as possible and be involved in determining the most suitable adjustments. The employer must not disclose any details to a third party about

Figure 5.1   Employee capabilities assessment.

The questionnaire is used to make a specific and objective assessment of the person's capabilities to determine if the working environment and working practices are suitable and sufficient or if reasonable adjustments need to be made. The outcome will help determine if a further analysis is required in the form of a risk assessment where specific hazards will be identified, risks evaluated and suitable controls implemented to reduce the risk of injury or harm.

DATE:	EMPLOYEE:	PERSON UNDERTAKING ASSESSMENT:

No	Capabilities	Suitable and sufficient	Unsuitable and insufficient
1.	Access into and egress from the premises		
2.	Manoeuvrability inside the premises		
3.	Signs and notices around the premises		
4.	Furnishings to include doors, handles and locks		
5.	Lighting levels – internal and external		
6.	Facilities (e.g. rest areas and WC)		
7.	Emergency warning signals		
8.	Evacuation routes and exits		
9.	Accessibility of emergency assembly points		
10.	Equipment required to carry out day-to-day duties		
11.	Written instructions, notices and safe operating procedures		
12.	Supervision levels		
13.	Allocation of work activities and duties		
14.	Manual handling tasks		
15.	Close support duties		
16.	All work areas and work activities		
Summary of assessment			

Risk assessment required *(circle)*	Date for risk assessment:
YES NO	
Review date:	Name of reviewer:

the person without his/her consent. When an employer is aware of an employee's disability, reasonable adjustments could be made as follows:

- Provide disability awareness training for all employees.
- Carry out physical alterations to the premises or workstations.
- Adapt or purchase suitable equipment.
- Adapt written safe operating procedures or provide in different formats.
- Ensure appropriate and adequate supervision.
- Allocate some duties to other people.
- Alter working hours and enable flexibility.
- Provide training or retraining.
- Transfer the employee to another role (if possible).

When deciding on the reasonable adjustments, consideration must be given to other health and safety factors. For example, if the adjustment would create another hazard or increase the risk level then the adjustment must not be made. However, the employer will need to show that the adjustment was unreasonable based on the factors mentioned previously.

Service provider

When determining whether you are providing reasonable access to your service, the following areas of the practice should be examined:

External approach
- Visibility of premises (signage identifying the practice)
- Distance and levels from car park to building
- Separating vehicle and pedestrian routes
- Accessibility from kerb to building
- Maintenance and lighting of route to building
- Suitability of car parking spaces

Can disabled people approach your building?

Entrance into the premises
- Colour of door against surrounds
- Step rises uniformed, colour contrasted and maintained
- Extended handrails on steps

- Positioning and adequacy of lighting
- Manoeuvrability at top and bottom of ramps
- Gradient of ramps
- Continuous handrails on ramps
- Height and operation of door controls/handles

Can disabled people enter your building?

Reception and waiting area
- Lighting and acoustics
- Junctions between floor surfaces
- Levels of reception desk
- Choice of seating and space for wheelchairs
- Appointment call systems
- Use of television/DVD and methods of communication
- Space and layout of areas
- Movement from one area to another

Are disabled people received fairly?

Internal areas
- Unobstructed corridors and sufficient space
- Level and temperature of heating appliances
- Colour of doors against surrounds
- Door controls
- Reflections, glare and lighting
- Stairs and handrails
- Signage and information
- Floor levels and surfaces

Can disabled people manoeuvre around the building safely?

Sanitary facilities (WC)
- Distance and route to WC
- Door contrast against surround
- Door controls and locks, outside opening
- Floor surface
- Size of area
- Visibility of fittings and grab-rails
- Accessibility of lights, flush, hand washing/drying and ancillary items
- Height of baby changing facilities

Can disabled people utilise your facilities?

Signage, information and communication
- Height of signs and notices
- Visual and tactile

- Clear, legible, easy to read against background including all practice promotional materials
- Pictograms
- Appropriate lighting
- Accessibility of information displays
- Appropriate verbal communication methods and disability awareness of staff

Do your communication systems convey appropriate information to disabled people?

Emergency evacuation
- Alarm systems – audible and visual
- Levels of evacuation – routes and exits
- Exit signs – include wheelchair symbol
- Means of escape from above ground level
- Escape plan for those needing assistance
- Escape routes unobstructed and well lit
- Safe distance from building achievable

Can disabled people evacuate your building quickly and safely?

All of the above-mentioned factors should be assessed to determine if your premises are accessible to employees and service users and reasonable adjustments made where necessary.

Access audit

Most barriers or obstacles to your premises and services can be easily removed and, therefore, can be relatively inexpensive. However, you may decide to enlist the services of a 'specialist contractor' to help you meet the legislative requirements and assess your premises. An access audit is an examination of the building, its facilities and services against set criteria to determine ease of use by disabled people. The access audit process is undertaken as follows:

- Initial consultation to determine business needs
- Detailed inspection of the premises covering all areas
- Investigation of areas used by members of the public and staff
- Priority areas identified
- Method of providing services analysed

- Report produced, detailing
  - □ areas of non-compliance
  - □ prioritised recommended course of action – reasonable adjustments

The access audit helps to demonstrate compliance with legislation, provides justification for the reasonableness of adjustment and improves access to the premises *(Source: Access Disability Ltd)*.

Summary

Dental practices must take 'reasonable steps' to ensure that service is accessible to disabled staff and customers. These steps should involve educating the team and raising awareness on disability issues, improving communication between the client and staff, changing policies and procedures to meet the needs of all clients or providing a reasonable alternative method of accessing the service. Providing ramps and other such aids could be way beyond the requirements of the legislation as it may not be deemed 'reasonable'. Dental practices are required to identify whether they are doing what is reasonable at present, and, if not, what steps need to be taken by balancing the needs of the organisation and those of the clients. People with disabilities do not have to reveal to you that they are disabled; therefore, you must ensure that everyone applying to or working for you or accessing your services is treated fairly. No person should be treated less favourably for a reason that relates to his/her disability. Employers are required to make reasonable adjustments to working conditions, the workplace and access to facilities and services to take account of the different needs of disabled persons.

Action – check the following

- Do your recruitment and selection policies and procedures encourage applicants with disabilities?
- Have you examined your premises or undertaken an access audit?

- Do you enable people with disabilities to use your services?

Frequently asked questions

Q. Can we refuse to interview someone for a position if the person has not revealed his/her disability in the self-declaration section on the application form?

A. Applicants should be encouraged to complete this section, with a supporting statement explaining the reasons for requesting the information; for example, 'to treat everyone fairly' could be used. However, the applicant does not have to reveal the disability; so, it would be classed as discrimination to refuse him/her to attend an interview. In addition, the applicant should be given the opportunity to apply for a position on his/her suitability to undertake the role and not the disability.

Q. The practice is a listed building and physically disabled people cannot access our services. I am told that I do not have to make any adjustments, is this true?

A. Listed buildings are not exempt from DDA. Firstly, you need to identify the physical barriers which prevent access and explore if there are ways of overcoming these by making reasonable adjustments. There are certain restrictions placed on the alteration of listed buildings – it is therefore advisable to seek specialist advice before starting any work.

Q. We are thinking about installing a ramp at the front of the practice. Is there anything we should consider to ensure this is done correctly and safely?

A. The law states that alterations can be made by removing the barrier, making alterations, avoiding the problem or providing a service or access by a reasonable alterative method, for example, by domiciliary care. Any adjustments made must comply with British Standards and Building Regulations. It is advisable to seek specialist advice to ensure that you are meeting the requirements.

Links to other chapters

Chapter 3 – Communication and training
Chapter 8 – Fire safety and emergencies
Chapter 17 – Policy
Chapter 19 – Risk assessment
Chapter 23 – Working environment

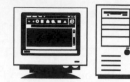

6 Display screen equipment

Scope of this chapter

- Introduction
- Legislation
- Definitions
- Possible health problems
- Analysing and assessing workstations
- Controlling risks

Figures

Introduction

Musculoskeletal disorders are often caused by poor ergonomics, which quite simply means the interrelationships between people, the workplace and the equipment used to carry out work. In practical terms, this means poor workstation design, incorrect posture, sitting in one position for long periods, repetitive movements or a combination of all four. With the increased use of technology in dental practices, staff are spending longer hours using display screen equipment than ever before. Most dental practices are computerised to some degree either in the clinical or office area or both; so, all dental staff are potentially exposed to the risks. However, it could be said that the level of risk in dentistry is relatively low because of the nature of the business and the fact that staff do not necessarily spend long periods of time at a computer workstation. Therefore, the legal duties placed on employers may not apply in dentistry. Although the risk may be quite low, it is important to consider any potentially adverse effects to ensure the health and well-being of staff while at work. This can be achieved by using a risk assessment approach to identify any problems and put appropriate measures in place to improve working conditions.

Legislation

- Health and Safety at Work etc. Act 1974:

    Employers have a general duty to their employees, so far as is reasonable, to provide and maintain equipment and systems of work that are safe and without risks to health.

- Health and Safety (Display Screen Equipment) Regulations 1992 (as amended):

  Employers are required to undertake a suitable and sufficient risk assessment on workstations used by 'users' or 'operators' and ensure that workstations meet basic requirements.

- Management of Health and Safety at Work Regulations 1999:

  Employers must undertake suitable and sufficient assessments of risks to the health and safety of employees and implement reasonable controls.

Definitions

It is important to have an understanding of the key terms used throughout the Display Screen Equipment (DSE) Regulations in order to determine if the regulations apply. The regulations require employers to ensure that all workstations meet certain minimum requirements by doing the following:

- Carry out suitable and sufficient analysis of workstations (risk assessment).
- Ensure that equipment provided meets legal requirements.
- Plan activities and provide breaks or changes in work activity to reduce employees' workload on that equipment.
- For DSE users provide, on their request, an eyesight test carried out by a competent person.
- Provide information and training.

The following key terms will help to decide if the regulations apply, in particular, with reference to **user and operator** and whether analysis and assessment of workstations needs to be addressed.

- Display screen equipment – any alphanumeric or graphic display screen
- DSE **user** – an employee who habitually uses DSE as a significant part of his/her work

- DSE **operator** – a self-employed person who habitually uses DSE as a significant part of his/her work
- Habitual use – continuous use for spells of an hour or more
- Significant part of his/her work – daily use of the DSE
- Workstation, the arrangements of equipment including the display screen and any accessories, office equipment, work chair and desk, work surface and the immediate surrounding work area

When deciding whether your staff are classed as users or operators it is useful to look at the following job examples which have been adapted from the regulations:

Definite users or operators:
- Secretary
- Data input operator
- Telesales/complaints/enquiries
- Librarian

Criteria – uses equipment continuously for spells of an hour or more, uses DSE daily, high dependency on the DSE and has little choice on whether or not to use the DSE.

May be users or operators:
- Receptionist (first example)
- Client manager
- Technical adviser

Criteria – may use equipment continuously for spells of an hour or more, uses DSE daily, may have high dependency on the DSE and has little choice whether or not to use the DSE.

Not users or operators:
- Receptionist (second example)
- Senior managers (infrequent use to generate statistics)

Criteria – does not use continuously for spells of an hour or more, does not use DSE daily, does not have high dependency on the DSE and has a choice whether or not to use the DSE.

The above-mentioned examples and criteria will help determine if you need to carry out a risk assessment as required by the regulations. To assist the process, ask the staff about their day-to-day work activities associated with the use of DSE. For example,

- Does your job role involve using DSE?
- Do you have a choice as to whether you use DSE as part of your job?
- Is using DSE a primary function of your job role?
- Do you use DSE every day?
- Do you use DSE for spells of an hour or more?

If the assessment shows that people do not come under the definition of user or operator it is still good practice to carry out some sort of assessment to ensure that they are working safely with DSE. The regulations also apply if 'users' are **working from** home or at another location.

Possible health problems

There are a range of health hazards associated with the prolonged and regular use of display screen equipment, although some are not recognised immediately as they occur over time. The hazards may be attributed to poor workstation design, the pace of work, unreasonable demands placed on employees to meet deadlines or targets and unsafe working practices. The most common health hazards are listed below.

Musculoskeletal disorders

Musculoskeletal disorders are usually brought on by a poorly designed workstation, prolonged use of DSE and an incorrect chair. The back, neck and arms are most commonly affected and this can cause swelling, discomfort and pain to differing degrees.

Work-related upper limb disorders (WRULDs)

Work-related upper limb disorders (WRULDs) are caused because the user sits in the same position for long periods of time, carrying out

rapid, forceful, frequent twisting and repetitive movements and adopting an unsafe posture. The arms, hands, fingers, wrists and upper body are most commonly affected, causing a pins-and-needles-like sensation, cramp and debilitating pain. A common form of WRULD is repetitive strain injury (RSI).

Eye and eyesight disturbance

There is no evidence that the use of DSE damages a person's eyesight; however, prolonged activity looking at the screen can cause visual fatigue. Poor lighting around the DSE, flickering of the image, poor positioning of the screen and illegibility of documents if copy typing can all lead to temporary fatigue, sore eyes and headaches. At the time of writing, a study is being undertaken in Japan, which indicates that there may be a link between heavy computer use and glaucoma. The results of the initial study show that further research is required in order to establish the validity of the research *(Source: BBC News)*.

Fatigue and stress

This may be caused by poor job design, poorly organised work load, working in isolation, unreasonable work demands or insufficient breaks. This affects not only a person's physical heath but also his/her emotional well-being.

Radiation and pregnancy

There is no scientific evidence of risks from radiation emitted by DSE. Similarly, there is no evidence that emissions from DSE can cause miscarriages. It is important to offer reassurances to expectant mothers and if they are unduly concerned, perhaps, finding alternative duties for the remainder of the pregnancy could be an option.

Skin rashes

This is usually associated with a dry atmosphere in the room/area where DSE is being used.

There may also be other pieces of electrical equipment in the area which add to the problem. The rash normally appears on the face and is quite simply rectified by improving the humidity which will relieve the symptoms and the rash will disappear.

Analysing and assessing workstations

If you identified that your staff are classed as users or operators then the law requires you to undertake a risk assessment of the workstation and put measures in place to reduce risks. However, even if you do not fall under the requirements of the regulations it is good practice to carry out some sort of assessment to ensure that safe working practices exist.

Assessment should involve the people using DSE and start with them answering a self-assessment questionnaire about their working practices (Figure 6.1). The outcome of this will help determine if further analysis and assessment of the activities needs to be undertaken. If no further action is required, the self-assessment should be kept in the personnel file and used for future reference, if required. It is good practice to monitor and review the assessment to identify any changes that may occur. Where the self-assessment identifies that further analysis is required or if employees are legally classed as users or operators, then a risk assessment must be undertaken. The risk assessment should address the following aspects (Figure 6.2):

- Display screen equipment (screen)
- Chair
- Other desk equipment
- Keyboard
- Desk or work surface
- Environment
- Software system
- Management
- Individual needs of the person

When the analysis and assessment have been undertaken, it will be necessary to determine the level of risk. The risk rating formula in Chapter 19 can be used to decide the level of harm, the likelihood of harm occurring and the overall risk rating. A decision can then be made on what controls are necessary in order to prevent ill health.

Controlling risks

If risks are identified from the assessment then corrective action is needed and controls must be implemented. When determining suitable controls an ergonomic approach must be adopted which requires the workplace, work methods and work equipment to be adapted to the person. It will be necessary to decide what is suitable and reasonable in the light of the situation. The result of the risk assessment will identify where measures need to be taken and their order of priority. Employees must be consulted with at all stages of the risk assessment to encourage commitment and to ensure that control measures are suitable. They should also be encouraged to report any concerns as soon as possible in order to prevent situations from getting worse. Where five or more people are employed the Management of Health and Safety at Work Regulations requires employers to record the significant findings of risk assessments.

Summary

The use of display screen equipment in dental practices is now widespread and forms a significant part of day-to-day work. Employers should identify those who are classed as users or operators and carry out DSE assessments of risks so that the risks can be reduced to the lowest level possible. Employees play an important role in preventing health problems by analysing their work stations and activities, making adjustments and discussing any concerns associated with the use of DSE.

Action – check the following

- Have you identified those who are classed as 'users' or 'operators'?

■ Have your staff undertaken a self-assessment of their DSE activities?

■ Have you undertaken DSE risk assessments and put control measures in place to reduce risks?

Frequently asked questions

Q. Do the Display Screen Equipment (DSE) Regulations apply to laptops?

A. Yes, portable DSE, if used by an employee/self-employed to carry out his/her job role, is subject to the regulations, regardless of where that person is using it. It is sometimes difficult to organise the workstation and activities safely when using laptops. However, the employer should advise on how to avoid problems and ensure safe ergonomic working practices.

Q. Should foot rests be provided for receptionists?

Figure 6.1   Display screen equipment self-assessment questionnaire.

NAME OF EMPLOYEE:		DATE OF ASSESSMENT:
1. Height of chair can be adjusted	YES	NO
2. Back tilt of chair back can be adjusted	YES	NO
3. Footrest is provided if necessary	YES	NO
4. Sufficient space for postural change and adequate legroom	YES	NO
5. Forearms are positioned approximately horizontal	YES	NO
6. Space in front of keyboard to support hands/wrists during pause in keying	YES	NO
7. Wrist rest provided if necessary	YES	NO
8. Height and angle of screen can be adjusted	YES	NO
9. Screen is clear of reflection or glare	YES	NO
10. Image is stable and free of flicker	YES	NO
11. Screen is regularly cleaned	YES	NO
12. Screen characters are clear	YES	NO
13. Keyboard symbols are legible	YES	NO
14. Brightness and contrast easily adjustable	YES	NO
15. Working areas free of trailing cables	YES	NO
16. All equipment stable and well positioned	YES	NO
17. Temperature and humidity comfortable	YES	NO
18. Lighting adequate	YES	NO
19. Document holder provided if required	YES	NO
20. Surrounding area conducive to using DSE	YES	NO
21. Regular breaks are taken away from the computer	YES	NO

If you have answered NO to any of the above questions you may need to make adjustments to the workstation and work activities to prevent health problems. The results of this questionnaire must be discussed with your manager who will determine if a DSE risk assessment needs to be undertaken.

Figure 6.2 Display screen equipment risk assessment.

RISK ASSESSMENT NO:	DATE:		
NAME OF ASSESSOR:	LOCATION:		
NAME OF USER OR OPERATOR:	DATE SELF-ASSESSMENT COMPLETED:		

	Yes	No	Action Y/N
Display screen (visual display)			
Can you adjust the contrast and brightness of your screen?			
Can you easily adjust the screen swivel and tilt?			
Can you easily adjust the screen height?			
Is the screen angled away from reflections and glare?			
Is your screen image stable and free from flickering?			
Do you clean your screen regularly?			
Are characters on the screen well-defined?			
Does the screen easily move for correct positioning?			
Chair			
Does the chair swivel freely from side to side?			
Does the chair have a minimum of five casters easily moved?			
Is the chair comfortable to use?			
Is the chair adjustable in height?			
Is the chair back rest adjustable in height and tilt?			
Is a footrest available if needed?			
If the chair has arms can it move close to the desk?			
Other desk equipment			
Does the mouse move freely and is it comfortable?			
Are document holders provided if necessary?			
Does positioning of other equipment prevent over-reaching?			

(*continued overleaf*)

Figure 6.2   (*continued*)

	Yes	No	Action Y/N
Keyboard			
Is the keyboard movable and able to tilt?			
Are the symbols on the keyboard clear?			
Is the bottom of the keyboard at elbow height?			
Are the wrists straight when using the keyboard?			
Is the keyboard comfortable to use?			
Do all the keys work properly?			
Is the keyboard glare free?			
Desk or work surface			
Is there sufficient space around and underneath the desk area to work comfortably?			
Is there enough desk area in front of the keyboard to rest your hands/wrists comfortably?			
Is the desk surface of low reflectance?			
Is the height of the desk suitable for the person/s?			
Is the size of the desk suitable for other equipment?			
Is the desk strong enough for the purpose and free from undesirable movement (sagging/rocking)?			
Environment			
Is the temperature and humidity generally comfortable?			
Is ventilation adequate?			
Are noise levels appropriate to minimise disturbances?			
Do windows have blinds to prevent glare?			
Are lighting levels suitable with no reflections or glare?			
Is there sufficient space to allow a change of posture?			

Figure 6.2 (*continued*)

	Yes	No	Action Y/N
Software system			
Is the software suitable for the task?			
Is the software reasonably easy to use?			
Does the software provide error messages and help screens?			
Management			
If you normally wear spectacles, or have any eye problems, have you had an eye test within the last 2 years?			
Do you routinely take breaks from the keyboard at least once per hour?			
Have you received adequate information, instruction and training to enable you to set up your workstation correctly?			
Do you have any complaints or concerns regarding the use of DSE?			
Do you know how to report defects?			
Individual needs			
Do you experience any aches or pains in your upper limbs?			
Do you experience neck/back/headaches regularly at work?			
Do you have any individual needs that need attention?			

Any other comments:

Hazard rate	Risk rate	Action priority
A Death, major injury, major damage **B** Over 3-day injury damage to property/equipment **C** Minor injury, minor damage to property	**1.** Extremely likely to occur **2.** Frequent/often/likely to occur **3.** Slight chance of occurring	**A1** – Unacceptable; must receive immediate attention before work continues **A2/B1** – Urgent; must receive attention as soon as possible to remove hazard or reduce risk **A3/C1** – Must receive attention to reduce risk **B2** – Should receive attention to reduce risk **B3/C2** – Low priority; reduce risk after other priorities **C3** – Very low priority; reduce hazard or risk after other priorities
Hazard rate:	**Risk rate:**	**Overall risk rating:**

(*continued overleaf*)

Figure 6.2 *(continued)*

Action in order of priority to control the activity	Date to be completed by	Date completed
1.		
2.		
3.		
4.		
5.		
6.		
7.		
8.		
9.		
10.		
Date for review of assessment:	Assessor signature:	

A. The risk assessment will help to identify if a person's posture is correct when seated at the workstation. The chair provided should be adjustable to accommodate a person's height and allow the feet to be flat on the floor with legs at a 90-degree angle. If this is not achievable then a foot rest may be required.

Q. Do we have to provide eyesight tests for staff who use computers?

A. The DSE Regulations place a duty on employers to provide eyesight tests for those who are classed as 'users' on the user's request. You need to determine who are classed as users. The information provided in the section titled 'definition' in this chapter will assist in identifying if any staff are users.

Links to other chapters

Chapter 3 – Communication and training
Chapter 7 – Electrical safety
Chapter 11 – Lone working
Chapter 19 – Risk assessment
Chapter 22 – Work equipment
Chapter 23 – Working environment
Chapter 24 – Working hours

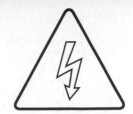

7 Electrical safety

Scope of this chapter

- Introduction
- Legislation
- Electrical hazards
- Principles and practice of electrical safety

Figures

None in this chapter

Introduction

Approximately 1000 accidents a year involving electricity are reported to the Health and Safety Executive (HSE), of which 30 are fatal. About 25% of these accidents are attributed to the use of portable electrical appliances and, according to the HSE, could have been prevented. These figures show that the use of electricity in workplaces presents many hazards, which, if not suitably controlled, can cause serious and permanent injury. Employers must ensure that electrical systems and equipment are installed, used and adequately maintained to ensure continued safety. Owing to the complexity and technical nature of the subject the information provided addresses the basic principles of electrical safety as it relates to the day-to-day use and maintenance of systems and equipment. The dental team should recognise the extent of their competence and know when to seek expert advice.

Legislation

- Health and Safety at Work etc. Act 1974:

  Employers have a duty to ensure, so far as is reasonably practicable, the provision and maintenance of plant and equipment that is safe and without risks to health.

- Electricity at Work Regulations 1989:

  Employers must ensure that all electrical systems, including high voltage to battery-operated equipment, is constructed and maintained to prevent the risk of injury arising out of work activities.

Managing Health and Safety in the Dental Practice: A Practical Guide, by Jane Bonehill   © 2010 by Blackwell Publishing Ltd.

- Provision and Use of Work Equipment Regulations 1998 (PUWER):

  Employers are required to provide and maintain safe systems and equipment and safe working procedures to ensure that work is carried out safely.

- Workplace (Health, Safety and Welfare) Regulations 1992:

  The workplace and the equipment, devices and systems shall be maintained in an efficient state, in efficient working order and in good repair.

- Management of Health and Safety at Work Regulations 1999:

  Employers must undertake suitable and sufficient assessments of risks to the health and safety of employees and others who may be affected and determine what measures should be taken to comply with duties under other health and safety legislation.

- The Regulatory Reform (Fire Safety) Order 2005 (RRFSO):

  Employers, occupiers or owners of buildings will need to carry out a fire risk assessment to identify the significant fire hazards, evaluate the risks and put suitable and sufficient controls in place to reduce the risk of fire starting.

Electrical hazards

Hazard identification is the first stage in the risk assessment process; therefore, it is advisable to read Chapter 19 in conjunction with the information presented in this section. Although this section does not cover all the stages of risk assessment, it provides an overview of hazards which lead to failures and recommendations on how to control them. Most electrical systems operate at either 240 or 415 volts; any voltage above 55 volts should be considered potentially fatal. The primary hazards associated with the use of electricity in dental practices include electric shock, electrical burns and electrical fires and explosion; the most common are as follows:

- Damaged insulation
- Faulty cables, extension leads, plugs and sockets
- Unsuitable equipment for the operation
- Incorrect use of equipment due to lack of competence
- Defects not reported
- Inadequate systems of work
- Inadequate over-current protection, for example, fuses or circuit breakers
- Overloading electrical circuits, causing overheating
- Faulty or poorly maintained protective devices
- Flammable substances contacting with an ignition source
- Replacement of light builds and fuses on supposedly dead circuits
- Loose contacts and connectors
- Poor maintenance and testing

The above hazards have the potential to cause interruption and failure in the electrical supply and electric shock, which can have multiple effects on the body.

Principles and practice of electrical safety

Once the hazards have been identified, it is important to then determine what needs to be done to prevent the risk of major injury or death. This section will address fixed electrical systems and portable electrical equipment.

Fixed electrical systems

- Construct systems to prevent the risk of danger.
- Examine 'older' systems using a competent person to check they have not been degraded.
- Ensure all wires and cables are suitably insulated and protected.
- Earth electrical equipment where necessary or take other precautions where the system is not earthed.
- Check any joints or connections for suitability and adequacy.
- Protect against excess current by ensuring correct amperage, that is, 13 A.
- Provide a means of isolating and cutting off the power supply.

- Control the work of electrical contractors and ensure that there is an exchange of safety information.
- Guard electrical sockets by fitting plastic inserts or hinged flaps.
- Examine and inspect systems at no longer than 5-yearly intervals using a competent person.

Any person inspecting and testing systems must be competent, for example, possess the necessary knowledge and skills.

Portable electrical appliances

See also Chapter 22.

- Select equipment suitable for intended purpose.
- Examine all new appliances before being used.
- Train users on the dangers associated with electrical equipment, any particular hazards, safe use of equipment and daily routine maintenance.
- Maintain records of training for hazardous equipment, for example, autoclaves.
- Devise safe operating procedures for hazardous equipment.
- Obtain the operator manual from the supplier.
- Create a maintenance programme for visual inspection.
- Create a maintenance programme for formal inspection and testing (follow manufacturer's recommendations). The frequency ranges from 6 months to 5 years and should depend on the risks. However, it is an extremely good practice to have this undertaken every 12 months by a competent person.
- Maintain an electrical equipment register supplied by the contractor to ensure that all equipment is included in the maintenance programme.
- Avoid using long trailing extension leads which could create a tripping hazard or damage the cable.
- Avoid repeated flexing of the cable to prevent damage.
- Remove the use of adaptors and replace with more socket outlets.

- Ensure that appliances are not sited near water or accessible to children.
- Take faulty equipment out of service and label accordingly; if necessary, discard it.
- Transport equipment safely to prevent injury or damage.

Any person inspecting and testing appliances must be competent, for example, possess the necessary knowledge and skills.

A risk assessment carried out by observing people working will help you to determine if electrical equipment is being used safely. It will enable you to evaluate if you are doing enough to protect people from electrical hazards or more needs to be done.

Summary

Electrical equipment and systems must be safe to use; it should be inspected and tested periodically and appropriate training provided. It is the responsibility of everyone to ensure that they work safely with electricity.

Action – check the following

- Has your fixed electrical system been inspected and examined within the last 5 years?
- Do you have a planned maintenance programme in place for your portable electrical appliances?
- Have you assessed the hazards associated with electricity and implemented suitable control measures?

Frequently asked questions

Q. What is the purpose of the fuse in a plug?
A. Quite simply, the fuse protects the appliance by preventing damage from a power surge. If too much power travels through the circuit, the fuse will break and the circuit will be broken. A standard fuse is a single-use device and must be replaced after the circuit has been overloaded.

Q. How do we know if the electrician is a competent person?

A. A person is deemed competent if he/she has completed an approved training course that is recognised by the electrical industry. The course should include an assessment of the person's knowledge and skill and recognition of his/her achievement, for example, a certificate of competence. The level of competence must be relevant to the work the person is undertaking. Nobody should carry out work if that person does not have the knowledge or skill to perform safely.

Links to other chapters

Chapter 8 – Fire safety and emergencies
Chapter 14 – Medical emergencies
Chapter 19 – Risk assessment
Chapter 22 – Work equipment
Chapter 23 – Working environment

8 Fire safety and emergencies

Scope of this chapter

- Introduction
- Legislation
- Types of emergency
- Emergency plan
- Fire safety duties
- Fire risk assessment

Figures

Figure 8.1 – Fire risk assessment record and action plan.
Figure 8.2 – The fire triangle.
Figure 8.3 – Fire protection inspection weekly record.
Figure 8.4 – Fire safety audit.
Figure 8.5 – Fire drill log.

Introduction

The consequences of fire and other emergencies can have a devastating physical and psychological effect on those who are directly involved. In addition, it can also have an impact on their immediate family as a result of human suffering and financial loss. The consequences not only affect people but also seriously disrupt business operation and, in the most severe cases, can lead to business failure. Being prepared for emergencies is a vital part of health and safety management as it helps to prioritise emergencies and put preventive and protective measures in place. This chapter will provide, in detail, specific fire safety measures; however, the principles should be applied to all types of emergency situations.

Legislation

- Health and Safety at Work etc. Act 1974:

  Employers have a general duty to ensure, so far as is reasonably practicable, the health, safety and welfare of employees and others. This includes protecting people from fire and other foreseeable risks.

- Regulatory Reform (Fire Safety) Order 2005 (RRFSO):

  The Employer or 'responsible person' must take 'general fire precautions' and carry out other fire safety duties that are required to protect 'relevant persons' in the case of fire.

Managing Health and Safety in the Dental Practice: A Practical Guide, by Jane Bonehill © 2010 by Blackwell Publishing Ltd.

- Management of Health and Safety at Work Regulations 1999:

  Employers must make suitable and sufficient assessment of health and safety risks, including risks from fire. Employers who share workplaces are required to co-operate with other people and co-ordinate any fire safety measures.

- Health and Safety (Signs and Signals) Regulations 1996:

  Employers (Occupiers) have a duty to provide fire safety signs where risks cannot be eliminated or suitably controlled by any other means. Signs must contain both text and pictogram and employees must be trained so they are familiar with the instruction.

- Building Regulations 2000:

  Persons planning and co-ordinating new buildings or significant alterations to existing buildings must take fire safety into consideration. In particular, the structure, means of warning and escape, internal & external fire spread, and facilities for disabled people and the fire service.

Types of emergency

An emergency can happen at any time; therefore, it is important to identify what type of emergency may occur in the practice. The following list provides a range to consider:

- Accidents
- Medical emergency
- Threats to personal safety
- Power failure
- Gas leak
- Storm
- Flood
- Sabotage
- Bomb threat
- Pressure vessel explosion
- Mercury spillage and other chemical escape
- Construction work
- Asbestos
- Radiation
- Fire

Everyone should be involved in identifying emergencies within the practice. This helps to facilitate the development of an emergency plan, which is both relevant and appropriate to the individual circumstances and situations.

Emergency plan

Emergencies will require an urgent and immediate response in order to minimise the consequences. Emergency procedures should be planned and well thought out so individuals can respond quickly without having to rely on information from managers or supervisors. The emergency plan and associated procedures should be documented, communicated and practised to ensure that it is fully understood and appropriate to the working environment. When developing the plan, the following generic factors should be considered:

- Action to be taken by the person discovering the emergency
- Special responsibilities for people such as calling the emergency services, shutting down the power or coordinating the emergency
- Responsibilities of all other persons
- Warning systems and locations of fire extinguishers or isolating switches
- Evacuation procedures
- Location of escape routes and exits and assembly (muster) points
- Arrangements for evacuating vulnerable people, for example, disabled persons
- Arrangements for equipment to deal with the emergency, for example, fire extinguishers
- Procedures for meeting and cooperating with emergency services
- Information, instruction and training arrangements to implement the plan, taking into consideration the needs of employees, visitors, contractors and patients

The emergency plan should state when a situation is to be classed as an emergency and how the emergency procedure is to be implemented. It must also emphasise that no one should put themselves at risk and that the aim is to ensure, so far as is reasonable, everyone's safety.

Fire safety duties

Legal definitions

Throughout the RRFSO certain terms are used, which directly relate to the legal duties imposed.

Responsible person:
- The employer if any of the workplace is under his control, or
- The person who has control of the premises in connection with carrying out the business function (occupier)
- The owner, where the person in control of the premises does not have control of the business function

Relevant person:
- Any person who is or may be lawfully on the premises, such as employees or patients
- Any person in the immediate vicinity who may be at risk

The responsible person is not expected to carry out fire safety duties in respect of fire fighters as he/she cannot be expected to know how he/she will operate in the event of fire. Therefore, fire fighters are not classed as 'relevant persons'.

The 'responsible person' is required to ensure the safety of employees and anyone else who is a relevant person; the following measures must be taken:

- Observe general fire precautions – measures that
    - reduce the risk of fire and fire spread;
    - are in relation to the means of escape;
    - ensure the means of escape can be safely and effectively used at all times;
    - are in relation to fire fighting;
    - are in relation to fire detection and warning;
    - are in relation to emergency action including information, instruction and training and alleviating the effects of fire.
- Carry out suitable and sufficient assessment of fire risks.
- Apply principles of prevention that emphasise risk avoidance and, if not possible, risk evaluation.

- Make arrangements for managing fire safety to include the measures for planning, organisation, control, monitoring and reviewing of the preventive and protective measures.
- Eliminate risks from dangerous substances by substituting them for substances that are less dangerous. In the event of an accident related to a dangerous substance make additional emergency measures available.
- Provide fire fighting equipment, for example, extinguishers, fire blankets or sprinklers. In addition, provide means of fire detection equipment and fire alarms appropriate to the needs of the premises and ensure this is maintained in efficient working order by a competent person.
- Ensure that fire resistance fabrications in walls and doors are kept in good order and fire doors have appropriate seals and strips and closing devices.
- Provide a means of escape that leads to a place of safety, in particular, doors that open easily and in the direction of escape. They should be sufficient in number, be suitably signed giving clear instruction; emergency lighting should be provided where necessary.
- Have consideration for vulnerable groups who may need special measures in the event of fire – for example, disabled people, expectant mothers and young persons.
- Have an emergency plan and associated procedures in place in the event of serious and imminent danger (see emergency plan above).
- Appoint a competent person or persons (from within the organisation where possible) to assist the responsible person in meeting his/her duties and implementing fire safety measures. A competent person must have sufficient knowledge, skills and abilities to carry out his/her duties.
- Provide relevant information to employees and anyone working in the premises on the fire safety measures adopted by the organisation.
- Adequate safety training should be provided to employees when they commence employment and when anything changes, and routine refresher training should also be provided. Training must include regular fire drills and must take place during working hours.

- Where responsible people share buildings they must communicate and coordinate fire safety measures and cooperate with each other.

The above-mentioned duties relate to all workplaces; however, dental settings may not present the same level of risk as larger organisations or more complex occupations.

Employees' duties

Employees also have a duty to comply with legislation, which includes the following:

- To take reasonable care for themselves and other relevant persons
- To cooperate with their employer
- To report any shortcomings in the fire safety measures

Fire risk assessment

Before undertaking a fire risk assessment it is suggested to read Chapter 19, which provides definitions of key terms and a simple risk rating evaluation (Figure 8.1). The purpose of a fire risk assessment is to help identify the preventive and protective measures that are required in order to comply with legislation, and also to consider the safety of premises and ensure the safety of people. Risk assessments identify how fire may start and what needs to be done to remove or reduce the risk of fire occurring and if fire does break out, how to control the spread of fire in order to contain it quickly and effectively and what fire protection is required. Risk assessments form the basis of prevention and protection and are an absolute must in order to meet the requirements of the RRFSO, and subsequently put controls in place to protect people. The fire risk assessment process should be carried out in the following stages:

1. Identify fire hazards

Fire cannot start without the presence of three factors; this is often referred to as the *fire triangle* (Figure 8.2).

To reduce the risk of a fire starting, take any one of these away and fire cannot occur. You need to identify where the three sources are throughout the premises; possible sources are as follows:

Sources of fuel – anything that is capable of burning easily and is in significant quantities.

- Furniture fabrics and curtains
- Flammable liquids, chemicals and gases
- Cleaning products and aerosols
- Accumulation of waste products such as paper or clinical waste
- Paper patient records, paper towels and so on

Sources of ignition – any heat source that is capable of setting fire to the fuel.

- Naked flames, for example, bunsen burners, matches and candles
- Electrical, gas- or oil-filled heaters
- Cooking appliances
- Static electricity and electrical equipment
- Faulty or damaged electrical equipment
- Sparks from cutting or soldering (relevance to dental technology)
- Arson

Sources of oxygen – capable of adding energy to the fire once started.

- Present in the air at all times

Additional sources:

- Oxidising agents – chemicals can react and cause the release of oxygen
- Piped oxygen and cylinders
- Ventilation and air conditioning systems

When identifying the above hazards look at all areas in the building, even those which are not routinely used, such as storage areas.

2. Identify who might be at risk

When identifying who might be harmed if a fire started, you will need to consider where people are located and situated at any given time. This will help identify why they are at risk.

Figure 8.1 Fire risk assessment record and action plan.

ASSESSOR:	LOCATION/WORK AREA:	RA NUMBER:
DATE OF ASSESSMENT:	DATE OF REVIEW:	

Hazard rate (HR)	Risk rate (RR)	Action priority (AP)	Overall risk rating
A Death, major injury, major damage **B** Over 3-day injury, damage to property/Equipment **C** Minor injury, minor damage to property	**1.** Extremely likely to occur **2.** Frequent/often/likely to occur **3.** Slight chance of occurring	**A1** – Unacceptable must receive immediate attention before work continues **A2/B1** – Urgent must receive attention as soon as possible to remove hazard or reduce risk **A3/C1** – Must receive attention to reduce risk **B2** – Should receive attention to reduce risk **B3/C2** – Low priority reduce risk after other priorities **C3** – Very low priority reduce hazard or risk after other priorities	

Hazards	Risk factors	Persons at risk	HR	RR	AC	Controls in place or required
1. Sources of fuel						
1.1						
1.2						
1.3						
1.4						
1.5						
1.6						
1.7						
1.8						
1.9						
1.10						

(continued overleaf)

Hazards	Risk factors	Persons at risk	HR	RR	AC	Controls in place or required
2. Sources of ignition						
2.1						
2.2						
2.3						
2.4						
2.5						
2.6						
2.7						
2.8						
2.9						
2.10						
3. Sources of oxygen						
3.1						
3.2						
3.3						
3.4						
3.5						
3.6						
3.7						
3.8						
3.9						
3.10						

Figure 8.1   (*continued*)

FIRE RISK ASSESSMENT ACTION PLAN:

RA NUMBER:

No	Control required	Target date	Monitoring date	Revised risk rating	Review date

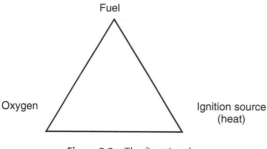

Figure 8.2 The fire triangle.

- Where the sources of ignition are situated in relation to the fuel
- Paper or other fuels stored close to heat sources
- Gas cylinders not stored securely, risk of falling over and damaging valves
- Waste allowed to accumulate
- Electrical equipment not being maintained
- If there is a risk of an arson attack
- Fixed electrical circuitry not inspected or maintained

Consideration should be given to the following:

- The location of staff at all times
- The location of patients, visitors and contractors at all times
- Special consideration may need to be given to the following people:
  □ Lone workers, for example, cleaners
  □ Disabled people (sensory or physical disabilities) including employees and patients
  □ Temporary/locum staff who may be unfamiliar with the premises
- Others in the immediate vicinity of the premises including neighbours

Consideration must be given to everyone including those who are not routinely present in the building, such as maintenance people.

3. Evaluate, remove, reduce and protect people from risk

Stage 3 is split into two key areas, preventive and protective measures. In fire safety, prevention means preventing people from being harmed, therefore, protecting them from danger. While evaluating risks, consideration should be given to both risk factors and control measures.

Evaluate the risk of fire occurring (risk factors)

This evaluation quite simply requires you to look at how fire might start and what is the likelihood, based on an analysis of the following risk factors:

Evaluate the risk to people from fire

When evaluating the risks to people the following should be considered:

- If a fire starts on the ground floor could it impair the escape route for those on upper floors?
- If fire starts in a storage area will people have to go past this as a means of escape?
- What is the possibility of fire or smoke spreading through the building via partitions, incorrect fire doors or doors being wedged open?

Once fire has started and it is capable of being sustained, it can spread very quickly throughout a building. Therefore, when evaluating the risk to people it is important to determine how fire may spread.

Remove or reduce fire hazard (control measures)

If possible, the hazards identified should be removed but if this is not reasonably practicable, then the risk from these sources should be reduced. The following are various ways by which this can be achieved:

- Ensure that furniture fabrics and curtains are of a fire-retardant material.
- Store flammable liquids, chemicals and gases away from heat sources and if necessary in a flame-resistant cupboard.
- Keep minimum quantities of cleaning products and aerosols.
- Improve internal and external waste storage and do not allow it to accumulate. Where possible, external storage should be at a reasonable distance from the building.

- Substitute flammable materials for safer alternatives.
- Replace naked flames.
- Ensure that a no smoking policy is adhered to on the premises including external areas.
- Replace portable heating appliances with fixed systems and ensure regular servicing.
- Ensure that all cooking, heating and work equipment is inspected and tested routinely and a planned maintenance programme is in place.
- Do not overload electrical circuits by plugging too many appliances into the supply.
- Provide electrical protective devices, for example, residual current devices (RCDs) and thermostats.
- Replace faulty or damaged electrical equipment.
- Implement a 'power/close down' procedure at the end of the working day.
- Take action to reduce arson by eliminating easy access routes into the building, keeping external areas free of debris and keeping outside storage areas locked when the practice is closed.
- Keep windows and doors closed where possible, in particular, fire doors.
- Store oxidising agents and chemicals away from heat sources.
- Ensure that piped oxygen and cylinders are inspected and maintained regularly.
- Store oxygen cylinders securely and keep stock to a minimum.
- Ensure that ventilation and air conditioning systems are checked and maintained regularly.

When you have removed or reduced the hazards you then need to determine how to remove or reduce the risks to people.

Remove or reduce the risks to people (control measures)

The above-mentioned control measures are aimed at preventing fire from starting. The next stage is to consider how to protect people should a fire break out in the premises. Protective devices are aimed at detecting fire, warning people, controlling the spread of fire and enabling people to get out of the building safely and quickly. The following should be considered in dental settings.

Fire detection and alarms must be suitable for the premises

Automatic detectors respond to smoke, heat or flame and must be located in appropriate areas. These range from single unit detectors to combined detection and alarm systems. Methods of raising the alarm vary from a verbal command, a simple bell or whistle to an electronic device which is operated by manual call points. Whichever system is used it must be capable of being heard throughout the premises and people should be familiar with the sound. The complexity of a fire detection and warning system will depend on the size and structure of the premises and the fire risks present. Advice should be obtained from a supply company on the type of system required to meet your specific needs. Detection and alarm systems should be tested weekly by a member of staff (Figure 8.3) and inspected by a competent person within the relevant period.

Fire fighting systems/equipment

There are two main methods of fire fighting – fixed systems and portable equipment. Risk assessment will help to determine the method that is most appropriate for your premises. Factors to consider are whether the hazards have been removed or the risks reduced to as low as is reasonably practicable and what risk remains. How long will it take for the fire and rescue service to reach the building and is there a good water supply for a fixed system? An example of a fixed system is automatic water sprinklers. Portable equipment consists of fire blankets and fire extinguishers. All cylinders are coloured red and display a **colour-coded panel,** as shown in Table 8.1, on the body of the cylinder. The size and number of extinguishers will depend on the fire risks in the building. They should be located where they are readily accessible, for example, near stairways, in corridors or landings and close to exits. The position should be clearly signed and stable to prevent them from falling or being inadvertently removed.

Figure 8.3   Fire protection inspection weekly record.

LOCATION:		DATE:		
INSPECTED BY:		**POSITION IN ORGANISATION:**		
Area/Device inspected			Yes	No
Fire detection system tested and in good working order				
Fire alarm tested and in good working order				
Fire alarm call points in good order				
Fire alarm call points signs in correct location and clearly visible				
Fire extinguishers in good condition and in correct location (visual check)				
Fire extinguisher signs and notices correctly displayed and clearly visible				
Fire doors unlocked and capable of opening				
Fire doors kept shut				
Fire escape routes free from obstruction				
Fire escape route signs correctly displayed and clearly visible				
Emergency exit signs clearly visible				
Fire action notices correctly displayed and clearly visible				
Emergency lighting in good condition and in good working order				
Escape routes clearly lit				
External escape routes free from obstruction				
Assembly point notice correctly displayed and clearly visible				
Assembly point accessible and free from obstruction				
Comments/Action:				
Signed:				

Table 8.1 Types and uses of portable equipment.

Type and colour code	For use on ✓	Do not use on X
Water [Red]	Wood, paper, cloth, plastics	Flammable liquids, electrical fires
Dry powder [Blue]	Flammable liquids, electrical fires	Metal fires
Foam [Cream]	Flammable liquids, paper	Electrical or metal fires
Carbon dioxide CO_2 [Black]	Flammable liquids, electrical fires	In confined space or metal fires
Wet chemical [Yellow]	Cooking oils, fats	Electrical fires
Fire blanket	Clothing fires, kitchen fires, waste bin fires	If the fire is not completely covered the blanket will not extinguish it

Portable equipment should be inspected weekly to check that they are correctly located, in good condition, are full and the test period is current (Figure 8.3). Extinguishers should be tested by a competent person within the relevant period. Table 8.1 describes the types and uses of portable equipment.

Means of escape

In the event of a fire, people need to be able to evacuate quickly and safely regardless of the size and structure of the building. An appropriate means of escape should give consideration to the following:

- Evacuation time – should be no more than 3 minutes in any building.
- Evacuation procedures – should be communicated and practised regularly.
- Location of occupants – consider all areas in the building, number of people likely to be on the premises at any one time, the physical and emotional condition of patients and their familiarity with premises. Special arrangements may be required for disabled people.
- Travel distance – distance from where the fire has started to the nearest final exit must be kept to a minimum. Remote areas of the building such as basements and attics must be assessed.
- Escape routes – everybody must be able to evacuate safely from any point in the building. Routes must be kept clear, doors on escape routes must be easy to open at all times and where doors are used in long corridors they must contain a vision panel. Stairs leading from basements or upper floors must provide safe evacuation aided by the use of handrails. Lifts, ladders and windows should not be used as a means of escape.
- Escape exits/doors – the number required will be based on occupancy levels, building size and structure and width of exits. They should open in the direction of escape where possible and not need the use of a key to open. They should enable people to proceed to the assembly (muster) point safely and quickly.
- Assembly point – must be clearly signed, accessible and located in a suitable area at least 12 feet from the building.
- External escape routes – if more than one escape route is required an external escape can be provided. This must meet special requirements.

Lighting

Escape routes must be adequately lit to enable people leaving the building to do so safely and quickly. In some buildings, natural light from windows may be sufficient; however, in autumn and winter this may not provide enough light. In addition, there may be some areas in the building where, if the power was to fail, it would be too dark to provide safe evacuation. In these circumstances, emergency lighting will be necessary. Consideration should also be given to external areas to allow people to proceed to the assembly point.

Signs and notices

In most premises, escape signs and notices will be needed. The results of the risk assessment will determine the need. They should be clearly visible, appropriately positioned and contain both text and pictogram. Signs and notices should provide the following information and instructions:

- Direction of escape routes
- Identification of fire doors
- Location of fire extinguishers and instruction on use
- Location of fire alarm call points
- Location of assembly (muster) points
- Action in the event of discovering a fire
- Action in the event of hearing the alarm

Mandatory signs are blue and safe condition signs are green. In some premises there may be the need for signs to be lit.

Fire service access

In the event of a fire, the fire service will need to access the premises quickly. Consideration should be given to vehicle access, mains supply and isolating services. To facilitate this a plan of the building indicating key facilities is a useful aid.

Monitoring, testing, audit and maintenance

All of the above protective devices must be inspected and tested routinely by someone in the organisation and this should be a planned process (Figure 8.3). As part of the overall management system, a fire safety audit should be undertaken annually to assess if the organisation is fulfilling the requirements of the Health and Safety Policy or if more needs to be done (Figure 8.4). In addition to this, a competent person should carry out tests and maintenance on protective devices as determined by the contractor.

4. Record, inform, instruct and train

Record the assessment

The significant findings of the risk assessment should be recorded as should the action to reduce risks. Where five or more people are employed this is a legal requirement. Figure 8.1 will assist in recording all the significant findings. Recording

the findings also helps to monitor the controls and assists in the overall review of fire safety arrangements.

Information and instruction

The employer (if he/she has not carried out the risk assessment) and employees should be informed about the outcome of the risk assessment and have the opportunity to consult on the findings. Their understanding of the process and any actions must be confirmed and their cooperation ensured. Staff must be informed about and instructed on any new working practices or changes to existing procedures. The risk assessment record should be made available to all staff and be readily accessible. Where premises are shared with other organisations the risk assessment must be communicated and actions coordinated appropriately.

Training

If the risk assessment has identified new working practices or changes to existing procedures, staff may need training to ensure that they are able to work safely. Fire safety training is an essential part of fire safety management and should be carried out during working hours. Fire safety training should be an integral part of a person's induction and take place as soon as possible after commencing employment. It should be undertaken as a continual part of employment, if job changes occur or in cases of non-compliance. Fire safety training should include the following:

- Fire hazards and risks and the action taken to control the risks.
- The emergency procedure should include
  - action to be taken on discovering a fire and hearing the alarm;
  - sound of the alarm;
  - location of alarm call points, escape routes, exit doors, assembly point and fire fighting equipment;
  - content of the emergency plan;
  - general fire safety measures.
- Evacuation drills should be carried out twice yearly and be recorded (Figure 8.5).

Figure 8.4 Fire safety audit.

General fire precautions	Yes	No
Have general fire precautions been taken to ensure the safety of employees?		
Have general fire precautions been taken to ensure the safety of others?		
Risk assessment	**Yes**	**No**
Has a suitable and sufficient risk assessment been carried out?		
Does the risk assessment consider vulnerable people?		
Has the risk assessment been recorded?		
Has staff been informed of the findings of the risk assessment?		
Has the risk assessment been reviewed?		
Principles of prevention	**Yes**	**No**
Have the principles of prevention been applied when implementing preventive and protective measures?		
Fire safety arrangements	**Yes**	**No**
Have the necessary arrangements been made to manage fire safety?		
Elimination or reduction of risks from dangerous substances	**Yes**	**No**
Has the risk from a dangerous substance been eliminated or reduced?		
Have emergency measures been considered to control an accident from a dangerous substance?		
Fire fighting and fire detection	**Yes**	**No**
Have appropriate fire fighting equipment, detectors and alarms been provided?		
Is portable fire fighting equipment accessible and indicated by signs?		
Are fire fighting measures suitable for the premises?		
Have persons been nominated to implement measures and have they been trained?		
Maintenance	**Yes**	**No**
Are fire-resistant fabrications kept in good order?		
Are door seals, strips and closing devices working and appropriate?		

(*continued overleaf*)

Figure 8.4   (*continued*)

Emergency routes and exits	Yes	No
Are all escape routes kept clear at all times?		
Do all escape routes lead to a place of safety?		
In the event of danger can everyone evacuate quickly and safety?		
Are the number, distribution and dimension of routes and exits adequate?		
Do all emergency exits open in the direction of escape?		
Are all emergency exits kept unlocked and are easily opened?		
Are all emergency routes and exits indicted by signs?		
Are all emergency routes and exits adequately lit?		

Vulnerable groups and special measures	Yes	No
Have special measures been made for vulnerable groups?		

Emergency plan and procedures	Yes	No
Have situations of serious and imminent danger been identified?		
Have appropriate procedures been established in the event of serious danger?		

Safety assistance	Yes	No
Have an adequate number of competent persons been appointed?		
Does the competent person have sufficient resources to fulfil their role?		
Has the competent person received training to effectively carry out his/her role		

Provision of information	Yes	No
Have employees been informed about fire risks?		
Have employees been informed about preventive and protective measures?		
Have employees been informed about the duties of the competent person?		

Training	Yes	No
Are employees provided with induction safety training?		
Are employees provided with training on exposure to new or increased risks?		

Figure 8.4   (*continued*)

Are employees provided with training as a routine and continual process?		
Does training take account of risks identified by the risk assessment?		
Is training conducted during working hours?		
Do employees rehearse a minimum of two evacuation procedures per year?		
Cooperation and coordination	**Yes**	**No**
Have the necessary persons liaised with each other to discuss fire risks?		
Has the responsible person taken reasonable steps to coordinate safety measures?		
Has the responsible person taken steps to gain cooperation from others?		
General duties of employees	**Yes**	**No**
Have all employees taken reasonable care for their own safety and that of others who may be affected by their actions?		
Have employees cooperated with the employer in meeting legal requirements?		
Have employees informed the employer of any shortcomings in fire safety measures?		

5. Review the assessment and revise if necessary

Review of the fire risk assessment should be planned and form part of the health and safety management process. Review may also be required where significant changes occur which could affect your fire safety measures as follows:

- Changes to the layout of premises
- Changes to working practices or work equipment
- Changes in legislation or professional good practice
- As a result of inspection or maintenance programmes
- Following an accident or incident
- As a result of the consultation process

If the above-mentioned changes identify that the risk assessment is no longer valid or sufficient it will need to be revised. Revisions should be recorded and staff informed of the changes.

Revisions must be monitored to ensure that they are suitable for controlling fire risks.

Fire safety policy

The completion of a fire risk assessment will help to identify if the practice fire safety policy is adequate or if there are shortcomings that need to be addressed. This is a reactive method of managing health and safety but will help determine if the fire safety policy contains sufficient detail or needs revising. The policy should show a clear commitment to fire safety and state who is responsible for implementing fire safety (specific and general responsibilities) and putting the arrangements in place to manage fire safety. The fire safety arrangements should reflect, in appropriate detail, the fire safety duties as listed in the 'Fire Safety Duties' section in this chapter.

Figure 8.5 Fire drill log.

DATE:	TIME:

NUMBER OF PARTICIPANTS PRESENT

Staff:	Visitors/Patients:	Other:

TYPE OF DRILL – SIMULATED OR ACTUAL:

Expected time of evacuation:	Actual time to complete:

PERSON IN CHARGE/COMPETENT PERSON:

Problems identified	Action required	Date action completed	Signature

Any other comments:

Date of next drill:

Summary

Good fire safety management is an important part of any organisation. The fire safety policy sets out the employer's intention; the risk assessment actively demonstrates the commitment. Together, these management systems and the preventive and protective measures in place will greatly assist in reducing the risk from fire.

Action – check the following

- Have you appointed a competent person to assist with fire safety?
- Do you inspect and test your fire safety devices routinely?
- Do you have an emergency plan detailing the action to be taken in the event of an emergency situation?
- Have you undertaken a suitable and sufficient assessment of fire risks?
- Does your fire safety policy demonstrate your commitment to fire safety?

Frequently asked questions

Q. How often should we rehearse evacuation procedures and should these be recorded?

A. Fire drills are recommended to take place at least twice a year. This helps to reinforce the action to be taken in the event of a fire and assists in identifying any areas for improvement. A fire drill log should be completed after every rehearsal and kept on file to assist with the fire safety audit and in case anyone wishes to see. The enforcing authority or insurance company may ask to see it.

Q. Should all staff be trained on how to use fire extinguishers?

A. The findings of your risk assessment will help to determine who should operate fire extinguishers. The use of extinguishers in an emergency situation must be well thought out and coordinated, so it may not be practicable to allocate the responsibility to everyone. When deciding who should have the responsibility, you should consider the safety of the person and ensure that the person does not put himself/herself at unnecessary risk.

Links to other chapters

9 Hazardous substances

Scope of this chapter

- Introduction
- Legislation
- Definition
- Anaesthetic gases
- Biological agents
- Chemical substances
- COSHH assessment
- Waste disposal
- Additional substances

Figures

Introduction

Hazardous substances are used and generated in all dental settings. They include chemicals used for cleaning, dental restorative materials and those produced by human beings in the form of bodily fluids. These substances have the potential to cause ill health if not suitably and adequately controlled. The adverse effects on a person's health may not be immediately recognised, but the consequences of injuries which do occur can be relatively major and long term. Controlling the use of hazardous substances is based on risk assessment where their use is analysed and appropriate control measures introduced. Legislation surrounding hazardous substances is both vast and complex. Therefore, it is the intention that this chapter will address those substances that come under the Control of Substances Hazardous to Health (COSHH) Regulations. Other substances listed in the scope as 'additional substances' will be given a brief overview as they are either not covered under COSHH or require specialist attention.

Legislation

- Health and Safety at Work etc. Act 1974:

  Employers have a general duty to ensure, so far as is reasonably possible, the safety and absence of risk to health in connection with the use, handling, storage and transport of substances.

Managing Health and Safety in the Dental Practice: A Practical Guide, by Jane Bonehill   © 2010 by Blackwell Publishing Ltd.

- Control of Substances Hazardous to Health Regulations 2002:

  Employers are required to assess the risks to health from exposure to hazardous substances by employees, the self-employed and others and so far as is reasonably practicable prevent or control exposure.

- Carriage of Dangerous Goods and Use of Transportable Pressure Equipment Regulations 2009:

  Employers have a duty to provide a safe place of work where a pressure receptacle is being used, to ensure the equipment is in safe working order and to design and implement a safe system of work.

- Chemicals (Hazard Information and Packaging for Supply) Regulations 2002:

  The supplier of the chemical must ensure that the chemical is safely packaged and properly labelled. He must also ensure that the recipient of the chemical gets the MSDS containing information to enable the user to store, use and dispose of the chemical safely.

- Control of Asbestos Regulations 2006:

  Employers must protect their employees, other people on the premises and other people likely to be affected by the work, against exposure to asbestos.

- Control of Lead at Work Regulations 2002:

  An employer must not carry out any work which is liable to expose an employee to lead until he has made a suitable and sufficient assessment of their health risks and the steps that need to be taken.

- Hazardous Waste Regulations 2005:

  Producers of healthcare waste have a duty of care to ensure that waste is managed appropriately from the point of production to the point of disposal.

Definition

A hazardous substance is defined as any substance which is capable of causing an adverse effect on a person's health. This includes chemical agents used, biological substances generated and any other substance which arises out of day-to-day activities. COSHH specifically defines hazardous substances as follows:

- Any chemical classified and labelled (orange square with a black symbol) under Chemicals (Hazard Information and Packaging for Supply) Regulations 2002 to include
  - □ harmful or irritant – label is St Andrew's cross;
  - □ toxic or very toxic – label is skull and crossbones;
  - □ corrosive – label is two horizontal dripping test tubes over a hand and workbench.
- Substances allocated a **workplace exposure limit** (WEL) as listed in the Health and Safety Executive (HSE) publication EH40, for example, nitrous oxide
- Substantial quantity of dust (may have relevance to dental laboratories)
- Biological agent, for example, bacteria and viruses

Workplace exposure limits (WELs) apply to substances that are airborne and therefore can be inhaled. The limit refers to the amount of substance in the atmosphere as a proportion of the amount of clean air. The lower the limit the more hazardous the substance. For example, a substance with a WEL of 1 ppm is more hazardous than one with 20 ppm. The limit stated in the regulations must not be exceeded. The WEL can be found on the material safety data sheet (MSDS) which the supplier is legally required to provide. A WEL does not apply to substances that can be ingested, injected or absorbed through the skin.

Anaesthetic gases

Anaesthetic gases which are used in dentistry include oxygen and nitrous oxide (N_2O). N_2O is a substance that has a WEL of 100 ppm as assigned by the HSE. The two main hazards associated with the gases as a

substance, rather than with the equipment, are as follows:

- Gas escaping from leaking valves
- Exhaled gas in the atmosphere

The use of anaesthetic gases must be managed in order to reduce the risk of exposure to dental personnel and anyone else who may be affected. Risks should be controlled by the following means:

- Use the minimum effective dose of N$_2$O on all occasions.
- Use an effective gas scavenging unit to trap waste gases and disperse them into the outside atmosphere.
- Ensure sufficient ventilation. For example,
  - General ventilation, for example, open windows or doors to assist dilution of gases
  - Local ventilation, for example, an extractor fan placed low on the wall or floor or air vents
- Use different size face masks to ensure they fit each patient.
- Train staff on the risks associated with the use of gases and the safety of cylinders.
- Monitor airborne concentrations of waste gas by sampling and measuring.
- Discourage patients from talking to reduce the amount of exhaled gas.
- Switch off machine when not in use.
- Prevent cylinders from falling over such that valves cannot be damaged.
- Check equipment prior to use to ensure equipment is not leaking.
- Reduce the need to lift and move cylinders to prevent damage from dropping.

Cylinders must be removed from the practice by a licensed company as this ensures safe transport and disposal to prevent inadvertent release into the environment.

Biological agents

Dental staff are exposed to biological agents as part of their everyday working life. The risk of exposure is incidental as it arises from the work undertaken. Risks from these agents must be controlled in order to prevent the transmission of infection. Chapter 10 specifically addresses the requirements laid down under the *Health Technical Memorandum* of the Department of Health (DOH HTM) guidance. Biological agents are classified as types and listed as four hazard groups. This is an approved list made under the Health and Safety at Work etc. Act 1974 and COSHH Regulations which impose requirements on employers to control risks. The four classifications and groups are as follows (*Source: HSE*):

- **Classification**
  - Bacteria
  - Viruses
  - Parasites
  - Fungi
- **Hazard Group 1** – This group is unlikely to cause human disease.
- **Hazard Group 2** – This group can cause human disease and may be a hazard to employees but is unlikely to spread to the community and there is usually an effective prophylaxis or treatment available.
  - Example – herpes virus varicella zoster, influenza type A, B and C and *Clostridium botulinum* (Botox)
- **Hazard Group 3** – This group can cause severe human disease and may be a serious hazard to employees. It may spread to the community, but there is usually an effective prophylaxis or treatment available.
  - Example – hepatitis B, C and D and tuberculosis
- **Hazard Group 4** – This group causes severe human disease and is a serious hazard to employees. It is likely to spread to the community and there is usually no effective prophylaxis or treatment available.

Hazard group control

Each hazard group requires the agent to be contained in the first instance and additional precautions introduced. However, in certain circumstances 'strict' containment measures may not apply because of the nature of the work or the nature of the biological agent. Risk assessments of work activities will assist in determining what level of control or containment is required to prevent the risk of transmission. Containment and control measures are discussed in COSHH assessment Steps 3 to 7 below. In particular, an immunisation programme must be implemented for all dental personnel.

Botox

A number of dental practices are providing non-surgical cosmetic treatment; one particular treatment is the use of Botox to smooth frown lines and wrinkles. Botox is the trade name for Botulinum toxin Type A which is derived from the bacteria *C. botulinum*. Botox must be managed in the same way as any other hazardous substance.

Chemical substances

COSHH requires all chemical substances to be used, handled, stored, disposed of and transported safely and without risk to a person's health. This applies to all substances that are classified and labelled as stated in the 'Definition' section earlier. Some chemicals used in dental practices have been assigned a 'risk phrase' which appears in the MSDS. Risk phrase refers to how the chemical reacts when exposed to certain conditions or special risks which the chemical presents. Chemicals of particular relevance to women of child-bearing age and new and expectant mothers are as follows:

- R40 – may provide limited evidence of a carcinogenic effect.
- R45 – may cause cancer.
- R46 – may cause heritable genetic damage.
- R61 – may cause harm to the unborn child.
- R63 – may cause possible risk of harm to the unborn child.
- R64 – may cause harm to breastfed babies.

An example of a chemical with a risk phrase is eugenol. Risk phrases assigned to this substance are 22–36/37/38–42/43.

In addition to 'risk phrases', chemicals will contain a 'safety phrase' which provides advice and describes the measures that must be taken in order to control exposure. For example, eugenol contains safety phrases: S26–S36.

It is important to obtain the MSDS from the supplier when carrying out a COSHH assessment to ensure that any special requirements are identified and controls implemented.

Amalgam

Where mercury is used, an assessment must be undertaken to determine the level of exposure and associated risks. The assessment should take into consideration the preparation of amalgam (e.g. mercury and alloy mixed or capsules); the environmental contamination; storage of mercury; waste amalgam and spent capsules and any special considerations for certain people such as expectant mothers and those with an allergy to mercury. Suitable control measures should then be determined as identified by the assessment (see COSHH assessment Steps 3 to 7 below). Amalgam waste should be stored in the regulated container under a mercury suppressant solution.

Amalgam separators

Amalgam separators should be fitted in all practices that use amalgam in order to meet the requirements of the Hazardous Waste Regulations. The practice needs to consider how many separators are required and where they should be placed. This will depend on the size and layout of the practice. According to Department for Environment Food and Rural Affairs (DEFRA), 'amalgam separators will need to be placed in such a way to protect all routes by which amalgam enters the drains'. Information from suppliers will assist in selecting the most suitable type of separator, where and how to install it and how to ensure it conforms to the British Standard.

Amalgam and mercury must be segregated and packaged in line with the regulations and consigned as hazardous waste. Amalgam has risk phrases of R23 (toxic by inhalation) and R33 (danger of cumulative effects) and safety phrases S (1/2), S7, S45, S60 and S61.

COSHH assessment

The risk associated with hazardous substances must be assessed and reduced to a level which is as low as reasonably practicable. A COSHH assessment is more than collecting data and filling in forms. It should clearly show that everyday activities have been assessed and suitable and sufficient control measures implemented. Before undertaking the assessment the following should be considered:

- Substances used during normal work activities, for example, dental amalgam
- Substances that arise out of normal work activities, for example, blood and saliva
- Information that may be needed to assist the assessment
- How the work areas and activities should be broken down
- Those people who may be more vulnerable because of individual circumstances or needs (see Chapter 3)

You should maintain an 'Approved Substance List' for all manufactured substances to assist with identification of substances and to facilitate review. The list should be updated accordingly and indicate substances that have been taken out of use (Figure 9.1).

The assessment is a systematic process which requires the involvement of everyone in the practice. In addition, it must be recorded where five or more people are employed. A COSHH assessment (Figure 9.2) is carried out as follows:

Identify hazards

This stage of the assessment should include the following:

- Make a list of all substances that have an orange warning sign or symbol (flammable, highly flammable, oxidising and explosive do not come under COSHH, but they still need to be assessed).
- Read the information label and leaflet in the packet.
- Obtain the MSDS from the supplier.
- Identify if a risk phrase has been assigned to a chemical.
- Determine the safety phrase given to the substance.
- Identify activities where biological substances pose a risk.
- Determine the hazard group for biological substances.
- Refer to the latest HSE EH/40 for substances with a WEL.
- Identify any other substance which could pose a risk to a person's health, for example, latex.

The above-mentioned assessment should be undertaken by talking to staff and observing how people work. The information gathered will identify what substances are present in the practice as recorded on the approved substance list.

Consider the risks

The next stage is to determine how the substance poses a risk to a person's health, how serious the effects are and how likely it is that people will be affected. The information gathered at the above stage will assist the process. Consideration of the risks should include an analysis of the following:

- The possible routes of entry into the body – inhalation, ingestion, inoculation and absorption through the skin.
- The effects of entry – severity of ill health, from mild acute to serious chronic must be considered.
- How people may be exposed – exposure may occur during the use, handling, storage, disposal or transportation and all factors must be considered.

- Who could be exposed – all groups of people must be considered including staff and others and, in particular, vulnerable groups.
- Exposure time – the length of time people are exposed to substances.
- Location – where the substance is used or generated as part of the work activity.
- Quantity – how much substance is used or generated as part of the work activity.
- Competency – what training have staff received and levels of competency.

- Existing controls – what existing control measures are in place and are they being used.
- The likelihood of substances causing harm or ill health based on the above analysis.
- Accurately assigning a level of risk to each substance used or generated.

The above risk analysis should be based on what is actually happening in your practice and will enable you to determine if your existing control measures are suitable and sufficient or

Figure 9.1 Approved substance list.

Name of substance	Supplier (including emergency contact)	Date listed	Date removed from use (see below)
Date removed from use: When a substance is taken out of use or is replaced by an alternative the date must be recorded to accurately reflect the substances in use.			

Figure 9.2 COSHH assessment form.

Name of assessor:	Date of assessment:	Assessment no:
Activity being assessed:	Substance assessed:	Location of assessment:
Hazard classification (label) or biological and hazard group:	WEL (EH40):	Risk phrases/safety phrases:
Persons exposed:	Vulnerable groups exposed:	Exposure routes:
Effects of exposure:	How exposure may occur:	Exposure time: (duration and frequency)
Existing controls:	Likelihood of harm/ill health:	Overall risk rating:
Additional control measures required (please specify)		
Elimination:	Substitution:	Enclosure:
Ventilation:	Reduce exposure times:	Safe working procedures:
Information & training:	PPE:	Rest and hygiene facilities:
Health surveillance:		Monitor or test controls:
Emergency procedure:		

COSHH Assessment Summary

Product name			
Manufacturer			
Hazardous properties			
Hazard classification	Toxic Flammable Corrosive Biological Irritant Harmful Other (please specify)		
WEL:	Risk phrase/s:		Safety phrase/s:
Appearance			
Used for			

Figure 9.2 (*continued*)

Used by whom				
Frequency				
Amount				
Adverse health effects				
Level of risk under normal working conditions	Very low	Low	Medium	High
Safe use required				
Safe handling required				
Safe storage required				
Safe disposal required				
Safe transportation required				
Personal protection required				
First aid measures required: Inhalation Skin Eye Ingestion Other				
Personal monitoring required				
Health surveillance required				
Staff training required				
Any other comments				
Planned review date:		Actual review date:		

The material safety data sheet (MSDS) must be referred to when completing this COSHH assessment.

if more needs to be done to control risks by determining additional controls.

Select control measures

If additional controls are identified it is important that the people exposed to the risks are consulted when deciding which controls to select. It is necessary to ensure that whatever controls are implemented they will reduce personal exposure to a level which is acceptable. To assist in determining the acceptable level, control of exposure is based on principles of good practice and includes the following:

- Design and operate activities and procedures to minimise emission, release and spread of hazardous substances by considering the following:
  1. Eliminate the use of a substance, for example, powdered latex gloves.
  2. Substitute a substance with one less hazardous.
  3. Enclose or isolate the activity or procedure, for example, automatic X-ray processor.
  4. Ensure adequate ventilation to minimise vapours, for example, air extraction unit (local) or open window (general).
  5. Reduce the number of people exposed and/or the duration and frequency.

6. Introduce safe working procedures, for example, ensure that areas are regularly cleaned and maintained, substances are stored safely and access to certain areas is restricted.
7. Inform and train all employees on the hazards and risks from substances and how to use control measures.
8. Provide personal protective equipment (PPE) where adequate control cannot be achieved by the other means shown above.
9. Eliminate eating and drinking in clinical or contaminated areas and provide suitable rest facilities.
10. Provide hygiene facilities such as hand washing sinks and appropriate barrier creams and hand hygiene products.

The above-mentioned principles are referred to as the *hierarchy of control*, which is designed to tackle the problem by containment (before the substance is released) or if not possible to contain, by controlling exposure. The hierarchy of control is used in descending order, that is, 1 is the most effective and 10 the least effective. Each control can be used in isolation or in combination with other controls.

- Account should be taken of all possible routes of exposure when developing control measures, for example, inhalation, ingestion, absorption and inoculation. There should be a recognition that exposure can happen through contamination of the general working environment, thereby exposing others who enter the vicinity.
- Control exposure by measures that are proportionate to the health risk. For example, more time and effort should be placed on managing the substances which pose a greater risk to health.
- Select the most effective and reliable control options to minimise the escape and spread of substances.
- Check and review regularly all elements of control for continued effectiveness.
- Ensure that the control measures introduced do not increase the overall risk to health and safety.

Use and maintain control measures

Once the controls have been implemented it is important to ensure that they are being used correctly and maintained in a clean and efficient working order. The following should be considered:

- If local ventilation is used it must be tested in line with the installer's instruction and records kept for at least 5 years (if required by the manufacturer/installer).
- Observe working practices to ensure that PPE is being used as instructed.
- Check that food and drink are not being consumed in clinical areas.
- Check that substances are being stored correctly and in line with manufacturer's instructions.
- Monitor cleaning schedules and ensure that areas are cleaned appropriately.
- Carry out routine checks to ensure that all controls are being used and maintained.

Monitor exposure

Personal exposure monitoring is normally required in the following circumstances:

- Where the assessment shows that there could be a serious risk to health
- If the control measures failed
- If the controls are not working properly
- If exposure limits (WELs) are exceeded
- **Specific reasons – if an employee's health record shows that health surveillance** is necessary (see Step 6 – health surveillance)

The results of monitoring must be kept for a minimum of 5 years.

Health surveillance

The purpose of health surveillance is to identify any adverse effects on an employee's health at the earliest possible stage to help determine suitable measures to prevent any further harm. There are no statutory requirements under COSHH to carry out health surveillance in dentistry because dental personnel are not exposed to the listed substances or processes. However, employers may decide to implement a health surveillance programme for reasons identified within the occupational sector – for example, mercury screening/testing by urine analysis and blood testing for vaccination purposes. If this is planned it should be stated in the employee's contract of employment. The frequency of surveillance is determined by a medical practitioner or after evaluating the symptoms a person is presenting with. Dental personnel are required to undertake an immunisation programme in order to protect them from certain biological agents, and records should be kept in order to monitor exposure.

Examples of an immunisation record and mercury screening record are included in this chapter (Figures 9.3 and 9.4).

Records

If health surveillance is undertaken COSHH requires the following to be carried out:

- Records must be kept for at least 40 years and contain the following details:
  - □ Substance exposed to and when (start date and frequency of use)
  - □ Surveillance test done and who carried it out
  - □ The outcome
- Provide HSE with copies of records on request and if the practice ceases trading.
- Allow employees access to their records.
- Allow employees time off during work hours for health surveillance.

The HSE recommends that personnel records should be kept for all employees regardless of the hazards they are exposed to, in particular for those

- exposed to toxic substances, for example, mercury;
- exposed to biological substances, for example, bacteria, viruses and so on;

- exposed to physical hazards, for example, ionising radiation;
- exposed to physical or mental stress.

Records should contain, at a minimum, the following details:

- Name, address, place, date of birth and gender
- National insurance number
- National health service number
- Job history, classified by job category

Pre-employment medical screening (PEMS)

It must be stressed that the overall purpose of pre-employment medical screening (PEMS) is to identify any specific measures that need to be taken in order to protect an individual from exposure to hazardous substances. Consideration should be given to the individual's specific health needs as identified on health records. PEMS must not be used to exclude someone from employment or to discriminate against him/her. In most cases, questionnaires are used to establish any individual health needs and include an explanation as to why the questions are being asked. If in any doubt about the use or wording of questions it is advisable to consult human resources or an appropriate advisory service.

Emergency procedures

It is important to be prepared in the event of an accident, incident or any type of emergency involving exposure to hazardous substances. The procedure should be appropriate to the assessed level of risk and meet the needs of the individual practice. In dentistry, an emergency procedure may be needed in the following circumstances:

- Spillage of a chemical, for example, mercury (mercury spillage kit)
- Blood or vomit spillage (appropriate chemical or vomit spillage kit)
- Sharps injury/inoculation from contaminated sharps (Figure 9.5)
- Fire caused by hazardous substance (fire plan and evacuation procedure)

Figure 9.3   Immunisation record.

Each member of staff must provide the employer with accurate and up to date information regarding their immune status. The information contained in this record must be kept confidential and only accessible to the employer, other authorised persons and the person it relates to. This ensures compliance with the Data Protection Act and Access to Health Records.

NAME OF EMPLOYEE: ....

JOB TITLE: ....

Vaccinations	Schedule	Date (approximately)	Evidence produced (please state)
Rubella (German measles) or see below	Administered during early teens		
Measles, mumps, rubella (MMR)	Administered during childhood		
Poliomyelitis	Administered during childhood		
Pertussis (whooping cough)	Administered during childhood		
Diphtheria	Administered during childhood		
Tuberculosis (TB)	Administered during early teens if a negative Heaf's test, BCG scar provides evidence		
Tetanus	Administered during childhood immunisation is temporary and may need to be repeated at intervals		
Hepatitis B	Recommended for clinical staff, course of injections followed by blood test. Status checked every 5 years and booster given if levels fall below 100 IU/ml	1. 2. 3. Blood test:	

I confirm the above record contains accurate and up to date information regarding my immune status.

SIGNATURE: .... DATE: ....

Emergency procedures are designed to address the situation immediately; minimise harmful effects; restore the situation to normal and inform others who may be affected. Staff must be informed, instructed and trained on the emergency procedures relevant to each situation. A significant event analysis should be undertaken, involving all necessary persons, in order to identify the causative factors and initiate changes to prevent recurrence.

Information, instruction, training and supervision

Employees must be given sufficient information, instruction and training on the following:

- The names of substances identified as being hazardous
- Risks associated with substances and the necessary controls

- How to use PPE/clothing
- Results of exposure monitoring and health surveillance
- Emergency procedures

It is important to ensure that the above information is fully understood by everyone. The method of disseminating information should be appropriate for your practice and, in addition, you should allow time for discussion and clarification on any points where necessary. Certain employees, for example, trainees, may need an increased level of supervision and this must be identified and acted upon.

Monitoring and reviewing risk assessments

Regular and planned monitoring should take place in order to check that the controls are being

Figure 9.4   Mercury screening record.

The COSHH assessment undertaken in this practice identifies that the employee is routinely exposed to the use, handling, storage and disposal of mercury. All reasonable measures have been introduced to contain and control exposure. Health surveillance through mercury screening testing is required to monitor personal exposure:

NAME OF EMPLOYEE: ....

JOB TITLE: ....

Date of test	Undertaken by	Outcome/results	Signature of employee

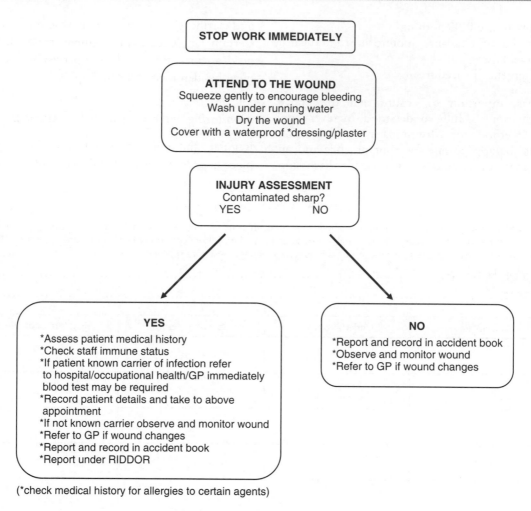

Figure 9.5   Inoculation injury procedure.

implemented, to identify any new risks and, if necessary, to amend existing controls. A review of the overall assessment should take place if any of the following apply:

- You suspect the assessment is no longer valid.
- The results of monitoring show it to be necessary.
- Work activities change or new substances are introduced.

Any revisions made to the assessment must be communicated to all employees.

Waste disposal

The Hazardous Waste Regulations place specific duties on waste producers, including dental practice employers, to ensure that waste is managed appropriately to prevent the risk of contamination to the environment, animals and people. Waste is classified as hazardous, offensive or hygienic and non-hazardous and must be colour coded, segregated, stored, disposed of and packaged according to the regulations. The Waste Management chart (see Figure 10.1 in Chapter 10) provides this information. Hazardous waste not listed on the chart includes the following:

- Fluorescent tubes
- Aerosols

These wastes should be placed in appropriate containers supplied by the waste collection company and labelled according to the instructions. Domestic waste is excluded from the regulations.

Storage of waste

Regardless of the quantities of waste produced, storage should comply with the following:

- Waste should be secured from access by unauthorised persons.
- Waste should be stored safely to avoid bags splitting or receptacles falling over and being damaged.
- Receptacles should be no more than two-thirds full and sealed appropriately.
- Waste should be labelled appropriately as instructed by the waste collection company.
- Areas/rooms should be kept clean and spillages cleared up immediately.

Practices which produce more than 200 kg of hazardous waste per year are required to register with the local environment agency. This figure is the total amount of hazardous waste from all sources. Practices are also required to keep the following records:

- Environment agency waste management license
- Waste transfer registration/contract
- Waste transfer notes/consignment notes

Some dental practices may be exempt if they are low waste producers.

The Carriage of Dangerous Goods and Use of Transportable Pressure Equipment Regulations 2009 place a specific duty on 'packers' of large quantities of clinical waste. The regulations require organisations to appoint a 'Dangerous Goods Safety Advisor' (DGSA) to be responsible for this function. However, it is unlikely that this applies to dental practices as the quantities of clinical waste will be below the requirement.

Additional substances

Asbestos

The risk to dental personnel from exposure to asbestos may be relatively low. It is therefore unlikely that the full scope of the regulations will apply to dental practice employers. However, all employers, owners or occupiers have a duty to manage asbestos by assessing whether asbestos is (or is likely to be) present in the building. Asbestos was widely used as a building material prior to 1999 when it was banned from use as a result of the consequences of exposure to asbestos fibres. If you work in a building which was built or refurbished before this time, then asbestos may be present in the premises. The Asbestos Regulations require the following:

- Assess whether asbestos is present – if you are unsure you may require assistance from a competent person.

If the assessment shows that asbestos is or is likely to be present, the employer will need to determine the level of risk that it presents. When determining the risk the following should be considered:

- How structurally sound is the building?
- When was any repair work last undertaken?
- What is the likelihood of structures being damaged accidentally or intentionally?
- Are there any planned repairs or refurbishment?

In addition to the above, a plan which identifies the affected areas must be prepared and include the following measures:

- The location of the asbestos and its condition
- How the identified risk will be managed

- Monitoring arrangements to routinely check the condition of the asbestos
- How the asbestos will be maintained in a safe condition or removed (it does not have to be removed)
- Providing information to maintenance contractors who may disturb asbestos
- Reviewing the plan to check that it is still valid and revised if necessary

If any repairs or refurbishment to the practice are planned which will 'involve' the asbestos, the following must be undertaken:

- A competent surveyor should be appointed.
- Possible exposure should be assessed to ascertain the type of asbestos, which is determined through sampling, the nature and degree of exposure and the required control measures.
- Assessments should be regularly reviewed and revised if necessary.
- A plan should be drawn up, which specifies address of premises, nature of the work, expected duration of the work, asbestos handling methods, what is necessary to protect employees and what is required of decontamination equipment and any protective equipment for others who might be at risk.
- Licensing and notification may be required – the competent person will advise.
- Employees should be informed, instructed and trained in the risks of exposure to asbestos and the necessary precautions.
- Exposure to asbestos must be prevented or as a last resort suitable PPE provided.
- Control limits for asbestos must be adhered to at all times while work is being undertaken.
- Control measures must be properly used, cleaned and maintained.
- Emergency plans should be designed to deal with accidents, incidents and emergencies arising from the work being undertaken.
- Cleanliness, designated areas, air monitoring and analysis, washing and changing facilities and storage and labelling of asbestos waste must be included in the plans.

Asbestos and asbestos-containing products are banned from use. However, if asbestos is present in the premises, it does not necessarily have to be removed. If it is in good condition and there is no risk of it being disturbed, it can be left.

Latex

The use of latex products in dentistry has diminished over the years; however, dental practices still use latex gloves when treating patients. In addition, latex may be present in rubber dam equipment; therefore, this must be classed as a hazardous substance and a COSHH assessment undertaken. Some people are sensitive to latex products which can result in a condition known as *occupational dermatitis* or *contact dermatitis*. Other substances used in dentistry may also cause occupational dermatitis, for example, some irritants such as disinfectants, soaps, detergents and oxidising agents. The signs and symptoms of dermatitis vary from a mild skin rash to redness, flaking, swelling and blistering of the skin, sometimes causing itching and in extreme cases severe pain. Dermatitis can also affect the respiratory system through the inhalation of airborne particles. A risk assessment must be undertaken to determine the extent of the risk and the control measures which are necessary in order to prevent or control exposure. In severe cases, the advice of a medical practitioner should be sought in order to monitor a person's condition and aid recovery.

Lead

The Control of Lead at Work Regulations apply to situations where employees are exposed to lead which is likely to be inhaled, ingested or absorbed into the body. Therefore, it is highly unlikely that the regulations will apply to dental settings. The regulations make particular reference to the fact that women of child-bearing age and young people may be particularly at risk. The lead produced in dental settings is from dental X-rays in the form of lead foil and, while this presents a negligible risk, it is worthy of some consideration. Risk assessment forms the basis of the regulations and can be applied to the exposure to lead foil as follows:

Step 1 – identify the hazards
- Analyse the nature of X-ray processing and the duration of exposure.
- Determine the quantity of lead foil involved.
- Obtain information from the supplier of X-ray films.
- Observe how waste foil is managed.

Step 2 – identify who might be at risk and in what way
- Establish who is most at risk and identify those who may be more vulnerable, for example, dental nurses in training or those who are exposed more frequently.

Step 3 – evaluate the risk
- Determine the likelihood of a person suffering ill effects from exposure to lead foil while undertaking his/her duties, based on the outcome of Step 1.

Step 4 – implement control measures
- Carry out effective hand hygiene immediately after handling.
- Remove waste from processing equipment immediately and do not allow it to accumulate.
- Ensure eating and drinking areas are remote from rooms where lead is present.
- Provide information, instruction and training where necessary.
- Remove lead totally by switching to a digital system (elimination of the hazard).

Step 5 – monitor and review
- Check that the controls are being implemented, identify any new risks and amend existing controls.

As previously stated, it is unlikely that lead foil from X-rays pose significant risks to dental personnel. However, it is good practice to assess the risks.

Legionella

Legionnaires' disease is caused by the bacteria Legionella found in hot and cold water systems and other equipment, which is capable of releasing water in the form of sprays or aerosols. An example could be the three-in-one syringe. However, specific conditions must exist for the bacteria to form and remain present. General controls require water systems to be kept clean and temperature kept as low as possible to prevent the bacteria from forming. The subject of *Legionella* is vast and complex and so specialist help is needed to identify whether the organism is present and how to manage risks.

Summary

In order to prevent the risk of ill health caused by exposure to hazardous substances, an assessment must be undertaken. The assessment process is relatively straightforward and should involve all members of the team. It is important to remember that not all hazardous substances are labelled. In particular, those that arise out of day-to-day activities may not be labelled. These activities need to be analysed as to what substances are present and how they can be controlled.

Action – check the following

- Do your COSHH assessments reflect how substances are used, handled, stored, disposed and transported in relation to your practice?
- Have you reviewed your assessments in light of changes that have taken place or new substances you have introduced?
- Do you communicate the outcomes of your assessments to all staff?
- Have you taken all reasonable control measures to prevent the exposure to hazardous substances?

Frequently asked questions

Q. What does DEFRA stand for?

A. The Department for Environment Food and Rural Affairs (DEFRA) is a government department committed to addressing environmental risks with the aim being to secure a healthy environment.

Q. Do I need a qualification to carry out COSHH assessments?

A. In order to carry out a comprehensive and effective COSHH assessment, you should have an understanding of the hazards and risks presented by the substances. You need to be able to analyse how people may be exposed and determine the necessary control measures in order to prevent or control exposure. In summary, you do not need a particular qualification but you do need to be competent in the process.

Q. Where can I find out more information about risk phrases and safety phrases?

A. Your chemical supply company must provide the MSDS when you purchase the substance. The MSDS will indicate both phrases if applicable to the particular substance; a comprehensive list of risk phrases can also be found at www.hse.gov.uk/chip/phrases.

Q. Do we have to assess flammable and explosive substances?

A. Although these substances are not covered under COSHH, an assessment must still be undertaken to determine the hazards they present and what controls are necessary in order to prevent exposure. The Management of Health and Safety at Work Regulations and other relevant legislation require assessments to be undertaken. Therefore, any substance classed as hazardous or dangerous must be assessed.

Links to other chapters

Chapter 10 – Infection control

Chapter 15 – Occupational health and well-being

Chapter 16 – Personal protective equipment

Chapter 19 – Risk assessment

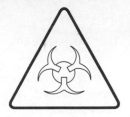

10 Infection control

Scope of this chapter

- Introduction
- Legislation
- Purpose of infection control procedures
- Methods of infection control
- Staff roles and responsibilities

Figures

Figure 10.1 – Waste management chart.

Introduction

There are a number of publications written by experts in the field of microbiology and infection control which are dedicated solely to this subject. There is very little point in restating that which is already written. Therefore, this chapter is intended to provide practical guidance on the implementation of the Department of Health's Decontamination Health Technical Memorandum 01-05, *Decontamination in Primary Care Dental Practices* (HTM 01-05); the

HTM forms the basis of this chapter. By 2011, it is expected that all dental providers will be registered with care quality commission. In order to meet the requirements of registration compliance with HTM is essential. The policy and guidance provided in the HTM is aimed at establishing a programme of continuous improvement in decontamination performance at a local level.

Legislation

- Health and Safety at Work etc. Act 1974:

  Employers must identify and provide, so far as is reasonably practicable, safe materials and substances and safe systems of work without risks to health.

- Health and Social Care Act 2008:

  Service providers must, so far as reasonably practicable, ensure that healthcare workers, patients and others are protected against identifiable risks of acquiring an infection.

- Management of Health and Safety at Work Regulations 1999:

  Employers to make suitable and sufficient assessment of risks to the health and safety

Managing Health and Safety in the Dental Practice: A Practical Guide, by Jane Bonehill   © 2010 by Blackwell Publishing Ltd.

of employees and anyone else who may be affected, and implement the necessary control measures.

- Control of Substances Hazardous to Health Regulations 2002:

  Employers are required to make an assessment of the risk of exposure to biological substances and where there is a risk to the health of employees or others, this risk must be controlled.

- Hazardous Waste Regulations 2005:

  Producers of healthcare waste have a duty of care to ensure that waste is managed appropriately from the point of production to the point of disposal.

- Department of Health – Health Technical Memorandum (HTM) 01-05:

  Healthcare providers have a duty of care to ensure that appropriate governance arrangements are in place and are managed effectively.

Purpose of infection control procedures

Advancements in disease identification have led to a recent review of health-care-associated infections and, as such, infection control requirements have altered. Up to date infection control procedures should be in place in dental practice to minimise the transfer of infections from person to person. It is essential that patients receive treatment in an environment that is as safe as possible and that all foreseeable risks are minimised.

Methods of infection control

The terms 'essential quality requirements' and 'best practice' are used within the HTM to define a level of compliance which is expected when the decontamination requirements are implemented. The HTM is intended to provide authoritative guidance to help dental practices identify areas for improvement, maintain acceptable standards and continuously develop their infection control systems and procedures.

Essential quality requirements

Essential quality requirements necessitate practices to provide a development plan which states how they will improve their decontamination processes. This will assist in demonstrating compliance to external bodies, for example, Care Quality Commission, Primary Care Trusts (PCTs) and Strategic Health Authorities.

- Instruments should be free of visible contaminants when inspected prior to sterilisation.
- At the end of the processing, cycle instruments should be sterilised.
- Instruments should be stored in such a way as to ensure that the risk of recolonisation is minimised.
- Practices should audit their decontamination processes at least quarterly using an audit tool compliant with local PCT policies.
- Practices should have in place a detailed plan on how the provision of decontamination services will move towards best practice.

Best practice

Best practice refers to the full level of compliance that may be achieved immediately or via a documented improvement from essential quality requirements.

- The cleaning process should be carried out using a validated automated washer–disinfector.
- The decontamination facilities should be clearly separate from the clinical treatment area.
- Instruments should be stored in a facility clearly separate from the clinical treatment area.

Policy

All dental practices should have an infection control policy in place which indicates full compliance with the essential requirements of HTM 01-05 and identifies a lead person responsible for infection control in the workplace. In addition, a written assessment of the improvements that the practice needs to make in order to progress towards meeting the requirements for best practice should be available together with an implementation plan.

The policy should be updated as legislation requires, or at two-yearly intervals, whichever is shorter.

Training

- Training and education in the processes included in HTM 01-05 should be part of staff induction programmes.
- Records should be kept of training and competency, and infection control should form part of the continuing professional development cycle required by the General Dental Council.

Cleaning instruments

- Prior to cleaning, reusable instruments to be cleaned should be segregated from items for disposal.
- Single-use device should only be used during a single treatment episode and then disposed of.
- Dentists should ensure that endodontic reamers and files are treated as single use regardless of the manufacturer's designation – in order to reduce the risk of prion transmission in dentistry.
- Reusable instruments can be cleaned using a washer–disinfector. For details of all operational aspects of using a washer–disinfector, follow the manufacturer's instructions.
- Hand-pieces should be lubricated according to the manufacturer's instructions.
- Hand-pieces that have not been processed in a washer–disinfector may require lubrication again before going into the steriliser.
- A separate canister should be used for cleaned hand-pieces and labelled accordingly.

Manual combined with ultrasonic cleaning

- It is important to ensure that the water/fluid is maintained, cleaned and changed at suitable intervals.
- The bath should also be kept free of dirt released during the cleaning process; good maintenance is also essential.

Manual

- Instruments should be cleaned in water at a temperature of 45°C or lower.
- Items should be fully submerged (if permitted in manufacturer's instructions) and scrubbed using a long-handled brush under the surface of the water.
- Water should be drained from the sink and instruments rinsed in a clean sink.
- Brushes should be single use. Where they are reusable, after each use, the brushes should be washed in hot water using the manufacturer's recommended detergent, in order to remove visible soil, and be stored dry and head up.
- To meet the requirements of best practice, practices should plan for the introduction of washer–disinfectors.
- At the end of the cleaning process, instruments should be inspected to ensure that the standards of cleaning achieved are visually satisfactory, that is, instruments are free from contamination, salt deposits or marked discoloration. The use of a simple magnifying device with task lighting may prove invaluable at this stage of the process.
- Instruments that cannot be cleaned should be discarded.
- Instrument processing should take place in an area separate from the clinical environment.
- Decontamination equipment including sterilisers should be located in a designated area with clearly identified dirty and clean zones.
- To comply with the essential requirements the designated area for decontamination may be in, or adjacent to, a clinical room.
- For best practice compliance a complete separation involving the use of a designated room will be required.

Sterilisation

A steam steriliser should be used for instrument decontamination. To ensure the safety of this device, the following points should be adhered to:

- Fill the reservoir daily using freshly distilled or reverse osmosis (RO) water.

- At the end of the day, cool and drain the water, clean and dry the chamber and leave empty with door open.
- Validation is necessary to demonstrate that the physical conditions required for sterilisation (temperature, pressure and time) are achieved. A competent person or service engineer will be able to ensure that validation is achieved.
- Carry out routine (daily, quarterly and yearly) periodic tests and maintenance. Store records of tests for each steriliser in a log book.

Cycle records

- If the steriliser has an automatic printer, the printout should be retained for a period of time determined by the profession or copied to a permanent record.
- If the steriliser does not have a printer, the user will have to manually record the following information in the log:
  □ Date
  □ Satisfactory completion of the cycle (absence of failure light)
  □ Temperature/pressure achieved
  □ Signature of the operator

Daily test

- The daily tests should be performed by the operator or user and will normally consist of
  □ a steam penetration test – Helix or Bowie–Dick tests (vacuum sterilisers only);
  □ an automatic control test (all small sterilisers) in line with manufacturer's instructions.
- These outcomes should be recorded in the logbook together with the date and signature of the operator.
- Before carrying out the daily tests, the user should
  □ clean the rubber door seal with a clean, damp, non-linting cloth;
  □ check the chamber and shelves for cleanliness and debris;
  □ fill the reservoir with freshly distilled or RO water;
  □ turn the power source on.
- If the steriliser fails to meet any of the test requirements, it should be withdrawn from service and advice should be sought from the manufacturer and/or maintenance contractor.

Decontamination areas

- Instrument processing should take place in an area separate from the clinical environment.
- Decontamination equipment including sterilisers should be located in a designated area with clearly identified dirty and clean zones.
- To comply with the essential requirements the designated area for decontamination may be in, or adjacent to, a clinical room.
- For best practice compliance, a complete separation involving the use of a designated room will be required.
- For essential quality requirements, layout of the decontamination area must ensure that dirty instruments do not come into contact with clean instruments and there should be a segregated in and out process.
- For essential quality requirements, there should be ventilation for input and extraction, sinks for washing and rinsing instruments and a wash-hand basin.

Hand hygiene

- Hand hygiene is an essential component of the infection control process and should be considered alongside the use of, not instead of the use of, gloves.
- Training in hand hygiene should be part of staff induction and be provided to all relevant staff within dental practices periodically throughout the year.
- Hand hygiene procedures should be practised at the following key stages in the decontamination process:
  □ Before and after each treatment session
  □ Before and after the removal of personal protective equipment (PPE)
  □ Following the washing of dental instruments
  □ Before contact with instruments that have been steam-sterilised (whether or not these instruments are wrapped)
  □ After cleaning or maintaining decontamination devices used on dental instruments
  □ At the completion of decontamination work
- Mild liquid soap should be used under running water when washing hands.

- Ordinarily, the hand-wash rubbing action should be maintained for about 15 seconds. After the exercise, the hands should be visibly clean. Where this is not the case, the hand hygiene procedure should be repeated.
- Hands should be dried using paper towels to minimise risk of skin damage and infection transfer.
- Hand cream, preferably water-based, should be used to avoid chapped or cracking skin.
- Fingernails should be kept clean, short and smooth. When viewed from the palm side, no nail should be visible beyond the fingertip.
- Staff undertaking dental procedures should not wear nail varnish and false fingernails.
- Rings, bracelets and wristwatches should not be worn by staff undertaking clinical procedures. Staff should remove rings, bracelets and wristwatches prior to carrying out hand hygiene. A wedding ring is permitted but the skin beneath it should be washed and dried thoroughly, and it is preferable to remove the ring prior to carrying out dental procedures.

Personal protective equipment

See also Chapter 16.

- The local infection control policy should specify when PPE is to be worn and changed.
- PPE training should be part of staff induction programme.
- Appropriate PPE should be worn during decontamination procedures.
- PPE includes disposable clinical gloves, household gloves, plastic disposable aprons, face masks, eye protection and adequate footwear.
- PPE should be stored in accordance with manufacturer's instructions.

Surface and equipment decontamination

- Surfaces and equipment used in the decontamination of dental instruments should be cleaned carefully before and after each decontamination process cycle. The procedure used should comply with written local policies.
- Wherever possible, surfaces (including walls, floors and ceilings) should be continuous and free from damage and abrasion. They should be free from dust and visible dirt.
- The ventilation system in the decontamination area or room(s) should be designed to supply reasonable quantities of fresh air.
- The use of carpets is not advised within any clinical or associated (decontamination) area.
- There should be coving between the floor and the wall to prevent accumulation of dust and dirt in corners and crevices.
- Cleaning specialist items of equipment (e.g. ultrasonic baths, washer–disinfectors, sterilisers and RO machines) according to manufacturer's instructions.
- Cleaning staff should be briefed on the special measures to be observed in cleaning of patient care areas or room(s) used for decontamination.
- The use of alcohol with dental instruments should be avoided.
- Cleaning equipment should be stored outside patient care areas.
- The patient treatment area should be cleaned after every session using disposable cloths or clean microfibre materials – even if the area appears uncontaminated.
- Dental chairs should be free from visible damage (e.g. rips and tears).
- Areas and items of equipment in the vicinity of the dental chair that need to be cleaned between each patient include
  □ local work surfaces;
  □ dental chairs;
  □ curing lamps;
  □ inspection lights and handles;
  □ hand controls including replacement of covers;
  □ trolleys/delivery units;
  □ spittoons;
  □ aspirators;
  □ X-ray units.
- Areas and items of equipment that need to be cleaned after each session include
  □ taps;
  □ drainage points;
  □ splash backs;
  □ sinks.
- In addition, cupboard doors, other exposed surfaces (such as dental inspection light fittings)

and floor surfaces, including those distant from the dental chair, should be cleaned daily.

- For blood spillages, care should be taken to observe a protocol that ensures protection against infection. The use of 1% sodium hypochlorite is recommended with a yield of at least 1000 ppm free chlorine. Contact times should be reasonably prolonged (not less than 5 minutes).

Water lines

- Water lines should be flushed for at least 2 minutes at the beginning and end of the day and after any significant period when they have not been used (e.g. after lunch breaks). In addition, they should also be flushed for at least 20–30 seconds between patients.
- Disinfection of water lines should be carried out periodically. In all cases, the manufacturer's instructions should be consulted.

Impressions

- Immediately after removal from the mouth the impression should be rinsed under clean running water until it is visibly clean.
- All impressions should receive disinfection according to the manufacturer's instructions.
- After disinfection, the impression should again be thoroughly washed.
- If the impression is to be returned to a laboratory a label to indicate that a decontamination process has been used should be affixed to the package.
- The responsibility for decontamination is that of the practice; cooperation and coordination of the process must be maintained between the laboratory and the practice.

Waste disposal

See Figure 10.1.

- Waste produced in dental practice should be segregated and disposed of safely.

- Each practice has a legal requirement to complete waste documentation accurately for the transfer of waste products.
- Waste documentation includes consignment notes for hazardous waste and waste transfer notes for non-hazardous waste.
- Waste is classified and segregated according to the waste type.

Immunisation

See also Chapter 9.

- Staff involved in decontamination should demonstrate current immunisation for hepatitis B and, subject to local policy, tetanus. Vaccination is considered additional to, and not a substitute for, other control measures.

Staff roles and responsibilities

Within HTM 01-05 a range of roles and responsibilities are described. It is possible that more than one of these roles can be carried out by one person. Each practice can establish its own system for managing staff responsibilities but must ensure that each responsibility listed below is allocated to at least one individual.

- **Registered manager:**
  This person takes ultimate responsibility for decontamination equipment ownership and the definition and allocation of the other responsibilities as listed below.
- **Decontamination lead:**
  This person takes responsibility for infection control and decontamination in the workplace.
- **Designated person:**
  This person acts as the interface between the practice and support services supplied externally.
- **Authorising engineer (decontamination):**
  This person plays an external role that provides guidance and advice on the compliance issues of decontamination.
- **Authorised person (decontamination):**
  This person provides technical support to the competent person and liaises with the authorising engineer.

- **Competent person (decontamination):**
  This person is responsible for the servicing, testing and maintaining of the decontamination equipment within the practice.
- **Competent person (pressure vessels):**
  Each practice will have a legal responsibility for the safety of its decontamination equipment, particularly the sterilisers that are pressure vessels.
- **Service engineer:**
  A person provided under a service level agreement or contract who is certified by the service agent or equipment manufacturer to be competent to both service and test specified decontamination equipment.
- **User:**
  This person has day-to-day responsibility for the management of the decontamination equipment and processes. An important function of the user is to ensure that anyone operating and testing decontamination equipment (i.e. an operator) is suitably trained and competent.

The registered manager should ensure that all personnel fulfilling the roles defined above should receive appropriate training such that they can demonstrate competency in their duties and that individual training records for all staff are retained. Training should always be supported by defined learning outcomes and competencies and may include, where appropriate, the following:

- An understanding of the whole decontamination process
- An understanding of their roles and those of others
- An understanding of the need for infection control and all relevant infection control
- Policies and procedures
- An understanding of, and an ability to perform, periodic testing where appropriate

Roles and responsibilities should be stated in Part 2 of the policy and be reflected in job descriptions.

Summary

The HTM provides comprehensive guidance on specific requirements for decontamination processes. All primary dental care practices should be looking to build on their existing procedures and bring them in line with the HTM standards. Care Quality Commission will be monitoring compliance against the standards in the near future. Practices will need to have a development plan in place to demonstrate that they are committed to reducing the risk of diseases being transmitted.

Action – check the following

- Have you communicated the content of the HTM to your team?
- Have you implemented a consultation process to enable the team to discuss issues and provide feedback on how to implement the requirements?
- Do you have a development plan in place to meet the essential quality requirements?
- Does the development plan include the identification of training needs in order to meet the required standard of decontamination?

Frequently asked questions

Q. Does the HTM require us to have a vacuum steriliser?

A. The HTM states that saturated steam under pressure delivered at the highest temperature compatible with the product is the preferred method of sterilisation for most instruments. There is no requirement to use vacuum type sterilisers unless the manufacturer of the instrument states this to be the case.

Q. Can we still use manual scrubbing to decontaminate instruments prior to sterilisation?

A. Manual scrubbing presents a risk of an inoculation injury to the person carrying out the task. In addition, it is difficult to validate that the instrument has been cleaned to the required standard. It should only be used when other methods are inappropriate for the piece of equipment or instrument as advised by the manufacture.

Q. We do not have any space in the practice for a separate decontamination area; does

Figure 10.1   Waste management chart.

Waste type	Waste classification	Packaging	Treatment and disposal
Clinical waste: Sharps Pharmaceutical waste	Hazardous	Rigid yellow sharps container	Incineration
Clinical waste: Soft clinical waste, infectious Body fluid contaminated items	Hazardous	Orange bag	Alternative treatment or incineration
Gowns, gloves, X-ray film, non-contaminated Feminine hygiene waste	Offensive or hygiene	Yellow and black stripe sacks	Landfill
Medicines Non-cytotoxic and cytostatic medicines including used and out-of-date stock	Non-hazardous	Rigid yellow leak proof container	Incineration
Amalgam waste Teeth with amalgam fillings – clinical, infectious amalgam and mercury – spent capsules, excess mixed amalgam, content of amalgam separators	Hazardous	White container with Hg (Hydrargyrum meaning liquid silver)	Metal recovery
X-ray fixer X-ray developer Wastes must be kept separate	Hazardous	Not specified	Recovery
Lead foil from X-ray packet	Non-hazardous	Not specified	Recovery
General business waste Packaging, cardboard, paper, food wrappers	Non-hazardous	Black sacks	Landfill, incineration, recycle

(Source: HTM 01–05)

this mean we will not comply with the HTM requirements?

A. Practices should be looking towards setting up a decontamination area that is separate from the clinical area. This should be incorporated into the development plan as part of essential quality requirements. If decontamination is taking place in the clinical area the risk to patients and cross-contamination of instruments should be assessed and risks minimised. Appropriate controls should be implemented as soon as possible, which reflect a risk management approach, in particular, clear separation of clean and dirty zones.

Links to other chapters

11 Lone working

Scope of this chapter

- Introduction
- Legislation
- Defining lone worker
- Risk assessment

Figures

Figure 11.1 – Lone worker risk assessment and action plan.

Introduction

The way dental settings operate and the demands placed on service providers have changed considerably over the last few years. This has led to an increasing number of dental professionals working alone. Working alone can create additional health and safety risks and employers are required to manage the risks that lone workers may be exposed to, just as they manage risks for all other employees. There are no legal duties to prohibit lone working; however, an appropriate safe system of work must be determined and communicated to the person/s who are working alone.

Legislation

- The Working Time Regulations 1998 (WTR) (as amended):

  Employers have a general duty to ensure that people who are working alone work appropriate hours with adequate rest and keep records to show that the regulations are being complied with.

- Health and Safety at Work etc. Act 1974:

  Employers must provide and maintain safe systems of work, which are, so far as is reasonably practicable, without risks to health, this covers the safety of lone workers. In addition employees must take reasonable care of themselves when working alone and not knowingly do anything that could put them at risk.

- Management of Health and Safety at Work Regulations 1999:

  Employers must undertake suitable and sufficient assessments of risks to the health and safety of employees and implement reasonable controls. *The risk could be increased because the person is working alone.*

■ Health and Safety (First Aid) Regulations 1981:

Employers should make an assessment of first-aid needs appropriate to the circumstances of the workplace and make available equipment and facilities enabling first-aid to be rendered. Lone workers may require first-aid training to satisfy this need.

Defining lone worker

Working alone refers to people who work by themselves without the support of their colleagues or without the direct supervision of their manager for a period of time. In a dental environment, this is most likely to include the following:

■ Cleaners who carry out their duties either before the practice opens or after it has closed
■ Practice managers who often arrive early and leave later than others because of business demands
■ Peripatetic staff who are mobile and travel to different sites
■ Personnel who work from home periodically
■ Domiciliary staff who work in someone else's residence
■ Dental technicians who often work in a laboratory on their own
■ Dental professionals who work on-site on their own, that is, access centre staff

Risk assessment

Under the Management of Health and Safety at Work Regulations there is a general duty to assess risks to which employees may be exposed. In the case of lone workers the risks may differ in nature. This involves identifying hazards associated with the work, considering the risk factors, assessing the level of risk and determining safety measures aimed at removing or controlling the risk (Figure 11.1). While it may be considered

that lone working is a relatively low-risk situation for the dental team, risk assessments should be conducted in order to ensure the health, safety and welfare of the lone worker and to put reasonable and appropriate controls in place.

Hazards to lone workers

The following points describe those situations which have the potential to cause harm in a lone working situation:

■ Personal security
■ Theft
■ Criminal damage to equipment/vehicles
■ Working in domestic/home premises
■ Environmental issues
■ Ergonomic/work space
■ Manual handling
■ Household pets
■ Road traffic
■ Medical history of lone worker
■ Remoteness of 'work place'
■ Access and egress
■ Isolation
■ Lack of close supervision
■ Working hours

Factors to consider when assessing risks

A range of factors should be considered to determine in what way the lone worker might be at risk and to what extent.

General factors

■ Can one person working alone carry out the activity safely?
■ Does the work involve going into known 'high risk' locations?
■ How often is work equipment transported and how may damage occur?
■ Is equipment awkward to handle or does it appear heavy?
■ If the lone worker was ill or had an accident how would the employer know?
■ Is it absolutely necessary for people to work alone?

Figure 11.1 Lone worker risk assessment and action plan.

ASSESSOR:	LOCATION/WORK AREA:			RA NUMBER:	
DATE OF ASSESSMENT:	DATE OF REVIEW:				

Hazard rate (HR)	Risk rate (RR)	Action priority (AP)			Overall risk rating
A Death, major injury and major damage	1. Extremely likely to occur	A1 – Unacceptable; must receive immediate attention before work continues			
B Over 3-day injury; damage to property/equipment	2. Frequent/often/likely to occur	A2/B1 – Urgent; must receive attention as soon as possible to remove hazard or reduce risk			
C Minor injury, minor damage to property	3. Slight chance of occurring	A3/C1 – Must receive attention to reduce risk			
		B2 – Should receive attention to reduce risk			
		B3/C2 – Low priority; reduce risk after other priorities			
		C3 – Very low priority; reduce hazard or risk after other priorities			

Hazards	Risk factors	Persons at risk	HR	RR	AP	Controls in place and is action required? (Y/N)
1. Alone in the practice						
1.1						
1.2						
1.3						
1.4						
1.5						
1.6						
1.7						
1.8						
1.9						
1.10						

2. Alone on domiciliary visits						
2.1						
2.2						
2.3						
2.4						
2.5						
2.6						
2.7						
2.8						
2.9						
2.10						
3. Alone working from home						
3.1						
3.2						
3.3						
3.4						
3.5						
3.6						
3.7						
3.8						
3.9						
3.10						

(continued overleaf)

LONE WORKER RISK ASSESSMENT ACTION PLAN:

RA NUMBER:

No	Control required	Target date	Monitoring date	Revised risk rating	Review date

Figure 11.1   *(continued)*

Working alone in the practice

- Is the practice open to public?
- Are valuables/money exchanged or held on the premises?
- Does anyone know the person is alone?
- What type of work is being undertaken and does it pose a significant risk?
- In the event of an emergency how will anyone know?

Home visits (domiciliary)

- Is the lone worker a frequent driver and familiar with a range of driving situations?
- Is the vehicle well maintained and serviced regularly?
- Do members of the patient's family pose a risk of violence or threatening behaviour?
- Is lighting sufficient to work safely?
- Is there sufficient space for the worker and any necessary equipment?
- Are the premises structurally sound and if using electrical equipment do installations appear safe?
- Are there any household pets and do they present a danger?
- Is the home in a remote area where access is difficult (e.g. rural areas)?
- Could the work/treatment endanger others in the patient's home?
- In an emergency situation is there safe evacuation from the building?

Some of the above factors will also relate to staff working from their own homes.

Working from home

- Does the worker take regular breaks?
- How does the employer maintain contact with the worker?
- How is the worker supervised in order to monitor any safety issues?
- Does the work activity affect members of the worker's family?

If the lone worker has an emotional or physical medical condition that would make it unsafe to work alone, the employer should consider if it is wise to allow him/her to do so.

The above factors provide a range of examples, but it is not an exhaustive list and there may be other factors to consider.

Risk control and safety measures

The aim of determining appropriate safety measures is to control the risks that the lone worker may be exposed to and ultimately protect that person from harm. There are a number of steps that can be taken, which will depend on the range of risk factors present. Risk controls should include the following:

General controls:
- Define what can and cannot be done by staff working alone.
- Provide information to the lone worker on the risks they are being exposed to and ensure that they fully understand the risks and the safe procedures to follow.
- Assess the lone worker's medical history and decide if the person is 'fit' to work alone.

Working alone in the practice:
- Identify significant hazards and analyse risks to lone workers and prohibit certain aspects, for example, manual handling activities, or restrict access to the public.
- Ensure that someone else knows the person is alone.
- Ensure that the worker telephones, texts or emails someone at arranged times and when leaving the premises.
- Fit a panic alarm that is connected to a staffed point.
- Provide personal alarms.
- Ensure that external areas are well lit.
- If leaving by car, park in well-lit areas.

Home visits (domiciliary):
- Identify known 'high risk' areas and carry out home visits to those areas only within daylight hours.
- Identify patients or their family members who are potentially violent and find out if there are animals in the house.
- Write to patients asking that animals be kept under control.

- Carry out manual handling assessments and provide information, instruction and training on safe handling techniques.
- Separate heavy loads or provide mechanical assistance.
- Substitute awkward/heavy equipment with items that are safer to handle.
- When travelling in the car remove equipment out of sight. For example, place it in the boot of the car.
- Keep a 'home visit recording log' in the practice for each staff member, for example, time of leaving practice, name and address of patient and the purpose of the visit. If there are any changes report to the practice.
- Have an effective communication system, for example,
  □ mobile phones;
  □ automatic tracking device;
  □ personal alarms.
- Telephone or text the practice when arriving at and leaving the visit.
- Telephone or text the lone worker periodically to monitor his/her safety.
- Provide travelling first aid kits.
- Inform staff that if they are in any doubt about their safety, work must stop.

Working from home:

- Carry out a risk assessment on the equipment that is used.
- Ensure that work equipment is regularly serviced and maintained.
- Monitor work activities by visiting to ensure that breaks are being taken.
- Communicate at arranged times by telephone, text or email.
- Devise a 'home working' policy which includes safe working limits, accident/incident reporting and what to do in an emergency.
- Provide first aid kits.
- Determine if it is reasonable for the person to work from home and consider how it may affect others in the home.

Summary

Employers have a duty to ensure the health, safety and welfare of employees while they are at work. The responsibility is the same for lone workers as for any other member of staff. Employers should identify situations when staff may be working alone and determine all the risk factors. Communication is an absolute must for lone workers. The employer should ensure that adequate and appropriate means of communication are in place. If any doubt exists about the safety of lone workers after the risk assessment has been carried out, then the activity should be prohibited.

Action – check the following

- Have you identified members of staff who are classed as lone workers?
- Do you need to carry out a 'lone working' risk assessment?
- Have you considered specific factors associated with lone working and controlled the activities by implementing safety measures?

Frequently asked questions

Q. Is it illegal to be working in the practice alone?

A. The law does not generally prohibit someone from working alone. However, the employer should identify the circumstances which could put the person at greater risk and consider suitable control measures. If risks cannot be suitably controlled then the person should not be allowed to work alone.

Q. During lunch time if there is only one member of staff on the premises do we have to do a lone worker risk assessment?

A. You need to consider what could put the member of staff at risk. For example, is the practice open to the public, do you have money or prescription medicines on the premises and therefore will this person be at greater risk because he/she is on his/her own?

Links to other chapters

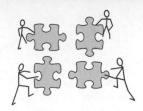

12 Managing health and safety

Scope of this chapter

- Introduction
- Legislation
- Reasons for managing health and safety
- Employer responsibilities
- Employee responsibilities
- Principles and practice of management

Figures

Introduction

It is strongly advised that you read this chapter in conjunction with Chapters 17 and 19, in order to develop your health and safety management system.

The overall purpose of health and safety management should be to implement the dental practice's commitment to health and safety as stated in Part 1 of the policy, 'General Statement of Intent'. This should clearly express your intention towards making the working environment safe and healthy for employees and anyone else who may be at risk from your day-to-day activities. In addition to Part 1, the policy should say who is involved in making this happen and their specific role and responsibilities and finally, the arrangements you have in place to demonstrate that you mean what you say, that is, how you will put your commitment into action. This will not just happen on its own. Like any other business function, health and safety needs to be managed.

Legislation

- Health and Safety at Work etc. Act 1974:

  Employers are required to prepare a health and safety policy statement of commitment and as often as may be appropriate revise the state-ment with respect to the health and safety of employees. In addition state the organisation and arrangements for carrying out the policy.

■ Management of Health and Safety at Work Regulations 1999:

Employers are required to have effective arrangements in place to manage health and safety. These arrangements must ensure the effective planning, organisation, control, monitoring and review of health and safety.

■ The Health and Safety (Consultation with employees) Regulations 1996:

Where employees are not represented by safety representatives under The Safety Representative and Safety Committees Regulations 1977, the employer is required to consult with employees on matters relating to their health and safety at work.

■ The Corporate Manslaughter (England, Wales and Northern Ireland) and Corporate Homicide (Scotland) Act 2007:

The organisation must manage or organise their activities in order to prevent serious accidents which could result in death of an employee, and will be guilty of an offence if a person's death amounts to a gross breach of a relevant duty of care owed by the organisation (employer) to the deceased.

Reasons for managing health and safety

All dental practices are subject to external pressures and forces of change – never more so than now. This has led to significant transformations in the structure of practices and how they are managed in order to meet the increasing demands. 'Managers' are faced with how to deal with the changes, provide direction to others and help people cope with the changing environment. An effective management system, which is people centred, will assist greatly in helping practices through the transition of change. Employees have a right to work in a safe, healthy and supportive environment, one that actively promotes the health and well-being of people and strives to ensure that this happens. Equally so, employees

have a responsibility to contribute; therefore, it is important that everyone understands the reasons for and the purpose of health and safety management in respect of their individual roles and the wider issues affecting the organisation. There are several reasons for managing health and safety but the following are probably the most recognised.

Legal

All of the activities undertaken in dental practices are subject to health and safety legislation. Employers and managers have a clearly defined responsibility and accountability for health and safety; therefore, they must comply with the minimum standards expressed throughout legislation. The results of non-compliance could lead to enforcement procedures which includes the issue of a legal notice or prosecution.

Moral

We have a sense of concern for our own well-being and that of others and we do what is possible to prevent the risk of injury, disease or harm. We do not intentionally carry out an action or omit to do something that could infringe on the health and safety of people.

Financial

The effects of accidents and ill health are staggering in terms of organisational disruption and the costs incurred. Some of the hidden costs are not immediately recognised and include sick pay, increased insurance premiums, repair or clean-up costs, replacement staff and damage to professional reputation. It is generally accepted that the costs of accidents and ill health far outweigh those of prevention.

Organisational

All dental practices have rules and acceptable behaviour standards that people must work within. These will be clearly stated in terms and conditions of employment, explicit in the Health and Safety Policy and enforced where necessary through disciplinary procedures. No organisation can allow employees to behave exactly as they wish.

Professional

Dental practices and dental personnel are expected to meet the requirements of the clinical governance framework by ensuring that the premises where dental care is undertaken are fit for the purpose. The General Dental Council (GDC) expects all dental professionals to put the interest of patients first and act to protect them.

Exemplar employer

Employers who demonstrate a commitment to the health, safety and welfare of employees will benefit by retaining a motivated workforce who recognise their responsibilities to health and safety and work as a team to achieve good acceptable standards.

Quality framework

A practice which has integrated health and safety management systems and procedures in place is able to measure performance against set goals. They are able to identify strengths and weaknesses and put realistic targets in place in order to achieve a desired outcome.

Health and safety management makes good business sense. It requires commitment from every member of the team and helps to reduce accidents and cases of ill health which gives everyone peace of mind.

Employer responsibilities

The Management of Health and Safety at Work Regulations 1999 state what is expected of employers in order to manage health and safety as follows:

- Carry out a suitable and sufficient assessment of risk to which employees and others may be exposed.
- Identify preventive and protective measures required by law in order to control risks; risk prevention principles required by law are as follows:
  - Avoid risk completely by elimination.
  - Where avoidance is not possible substitute with something less hazardous.
  - Combat the risk at source.
  - Adapt the work activity to the person who is undertaking it.
  - Use advancement in technology and best practice guidance and analyse the way work is organised in order to develop prevention strategies.
  - Look at prevention strategies that aim to protect everyone and not just one person.
  - Ensure information and instruction are clearly understood by all employees.
- Make arrangements for putting into practice the preventive and protective measures, in particular, planning, organisation, control, monitoring and review.
- Provide health surveillance that is appropriate to the risk identified in the workplace.
- Appoint competent person/s to assist with health and safety (if the employer has the necessary competencies and time this may not be required).
- Set up procedures to deal with serious and imminent dangers including having sufficient and competent personnel to evacuate people from the premises.
- Establish contacts with external emergency services, for example, the local fire service.
- Provide employees with information concerning the risks they are exposed to and how these are controlled. The procedures for serious and imminent danger, the identity of the competent person and any risks have been identified and notified by others sharing the workplace.
- Employers who share premises or workplaces must cooperate with each other, inform one another on the risks arising from their activities and coordinate health and safety measures.

- If another employer's employee is working in the premises, he/she must be provided with information on the risks they are exposed to, the control measures and the person responsible for emergency evacuation procedures.
- Health and safety training must be identified and provided to ensure that employees are capable of carrying out their duties safely.
- Locum/temporary workers must be provided with the necessary information in order to work safely. In addition, employers and self-employed persons must provide certain information to employment agencies before they start work.
- Risk assessment of activities for new and expectant mothers must be undertaken and the risk avoided where possible. If this is not possible the necessary controls must be introduced.
- If a new or expectant mother works at night and a certificate from a medical practitioner states that for health and safety reason she should not work those hours then she must be suspended with payment of wages.
- A new or expectant mother should be strongly encouraged to inform the employer in writing if she is pregnant, has given birth within the last 6 months, or is breastfeeding so that the employer can execute his/her legal duties.
- Risk assessments must be undertaken for young persons before they start work and activities prohibited where a significant risk remains which cannot be suitably controlled.

Leadership and commitment from the top should be clearly demonstrated, ownership of health and safety must pass through all levels of the practice and everyone should be held accountable for their actions. The next section explores the responsibilities of the whole team and describes their involvement in the management of health and safety.

Employee responsibilities

The management of health and safety is concerned with people at all levels of the dental practice. However, realistically, each person or his/her position within the practice will determine the actual involvement, role, responsibility and accountability.

Delegation of health and safety duties is an essential part of the day-to-day running of a busy dental practice; no one person can make all the decisions and do all the work. Delegation is, therefore, where one person gives someone else the control and authority to perform the health and safety function/s. However, if that person is expected to accept this control and authority, it is essential they have the ability and capabilities to carry out the role competently and safely. The delegation and acceptance of the role means that the person also accepts accountability.

Accountability must be understood by all members of the dental team, and each person should be answerable for his/her actions when performing tasks and functions. However, all persons in the 'chain of command' are still accountable for the delegation of the tasks; delegation does not mean accountability ceases.

We now examine a typical organisational structure and identify specific roles and responsibilities for health and safety.

Managing director, owner, proprietor or employer

Whatever title is assigned to this person he/she will have ultimate responsibility for business planning, safety policy design, development and implementation. The person at the top of the chain of command is accountable for his/her actions, will have overall responsibility and vicarious liability for health and safety and should sign the Health and Safety Practice Policy. This person will usually delegate the day-to-day running of the dental practice including health and safety management to a competent person, for example, the practice manager. It is important to consider, that where the employer/occupier is not the owner of the premises and or equipment certain duties are imposed upon the owner (see Chapter 23).

Practice manager

This person is responsible for carrying out specific health and safety duties. This includes ensuring that the practice policy is implemented and adhered to by all staff, safety procedures are adopted and equipment is used correctly to ensure safety; organising safety information and training; liaising with health and safety specialists for advice and assistance and ensuring that control measures are appropriate. The practice manager will also determine effective delegation of certain duties to others.

Other members of staff

All persons are responsible for carrying out their day-to-day duties safely and to report any discrepancies in health and safety arrangements. They must familiarise themselves with the contents of the Health and Safety Policy, be aware of updates in legislation that may affect their duties and act positively to instructions or warning signs and notices. Legislation states that all employees will have the opportunity to consult on health and safety issues, either directly by the employer or through other persons. This may require someone to be elected as the health and safety representative; however, it will be dependent on the size of the practice and number of people employed.

External people

Other people whom the practice is dependent on play a role in assisting with the management process, for example, hazardous waste collectors, delivery drivers and dental laboratories. These people must be clear on what are acceptable and unacceptable behaviours and working practices and cooperate by complying with the policy.

The Management Regulations places a requirement on employers to carry out risk assessment; this is discussed in detail in Chapter 19. The principles of risk assessment are embedded in the general principles for managing health and safety; the next section explores this belief.

Principles and practice of management

Most dental practices will be able to demonstrate a level of compliance with Health and Safety Regulations, essential quality requirements and good practice. This is a crucial part of health and safety management; it is the foundation on which the management system is built, but it is only the start. The next stage is to develop the system through a formal and structured practical management process. A practical management process should include an identification of which system is in place at the moment and what needs to be done to develop the system. A practical management process will assist in recognising results and focus on risk reduction, thereby adopting a risk management approach to health and safety. The following principles will assist in managing health and safety in all dental practices. These are based on the Health and Safety Executive's (HSE's) 'Five Steps to Managing Health and Safety'.

1. Developing a policy
2. Organising the team
3. Planning and implementing
4. Monitoring and measuring performance
5. Performance review and audit

Before we address the five steps in detail, you will need to determine how well you are managing health and safety at the moment. An 'initial status review' of your health and safety management arrangements should be carried out in order to identify your current situation. It must be emphasised that the purpose of the initial status review is to provide a summary of your existing management status and is not a comprehensive and detailed audit. The information gathered will help determine a course of action aimed at developing the health and safety management system (Figure 12.1).

1. Develop a policy

Successful health and safety management requires a Health and Safety Policy with specific objectives that influences all your business activities.

Figure 12.1 Initial status review.

Question	Yes	No	Action
1. Develop a policy			
a. Do you have a written Health and Safety Policy? *(legal requirement 5 + employed)*			
b. Have the contents of the policy been communicated to all?			
c. Is the policy up to date?			
d. Does the policy contain a statement of commitment to the health and safety of everyone?			
e. Does the policy clearly show who is responsible for what?			
f. Does the policy set out the arrangements for health and safety?			
2. Organise the team			
a. Do you have a system for communicating health and safety?			
b. Is competence assessed and training needs identified?			
c. Does someone take control of health and safety issues?			
d. Do you work together as a team to ensure health and safety?			
3. Planning and implementing			
a. Do you set health and safety standards that have to be achieved?			
b. Have risk assessments been conducted?			
c. Are the results of risk assessment communicated to all?			
d. Have you got safe operating procedures for 'at risk tasks'?			
e. Are risks adequately controlled throughout the practice?			
f. Is everyone actively involved in making the practice safer?			
4. Monitor and measure performance			
a. Do you carry out health and safety inspections internally?			
b. Do you act on the results of the inspections?			
c. Do you report and record all cases of accidents?			
d. Do you investigate all accidents including near misses?			
e. Do you take action to prevent further accidents occurring?			
f. Do you discuss health and safety at team meetings?			
g. Do you know how often equipment failures occur?			
h. Are you monitoring your health and safety performance?			
5. Audit and review			
a. Do you have a procedure for reviewing health and safety?			
b. Do you discuss the need for improvements?			

Figure 12.1 (*continued*)

Question	Yes	No	Action
c. Do you revise systems and procedure when necessary?			
d. Do you agree on any changes before they are actioned?			
e. Are all members of the team involved in the formal review?			
Action required			

NAME AND JOB TITLE OF REVIEWER:	DATE OF REVIEW:

The policy must be effectively implemented and should be an integrated part of the dental practice decision-making process. Organisations that employ less than five 'employees' are exempt from the requirement to provide a written policy. This exemption should not mean that a practice does not need a Health and Safety Policy as the policy demonstrates a commitment to health and safety. The policy should be reviewed periodically and revised if necessary and the revisions brought to the notice of all employees. When you have carried out the 'initial status review' you will then need to examine your health and safety policy in more detail to ensure that it contains the following information:

- Clearly defined statement of their intention from 'top management'
- A commitment to the health and safety of all persons
- Compliance with legislation, essential quality requirements and best practice
- Appropriate arrangements in place for the nature and scale of the organisation's health and safety risks
- Benefits of managing health and safety

- A systematic identification and control of risk
- Appropriate allocation of resources
- Involvement of all employees and other interested parties through consultation and communication processes
- Recognising changes and continually improving systems and procedures
- Periodic review to ensure that it remains relevant, current and appropriate to the organisation
- Allocation of delegated responsibilities
- Distribution of the policy to interested parties

The policy must be clearly written and needs to include the health, safety and welfare of all staff, patients, visitors and others whom you are in contact with. It should include a commitment to other bodies whom your business depends on, for example, Primary Care Trust.

2. Organise the team

Organising the team is about ensuring that you have an appropriate management structure in place which addresses health and safety at all levels of the organisation (Figure 17.3). Part 2 of your Health and Safety Policy formally details the organisational structure for implementing the policy and emphasises the responsibilities of individuals. To ensure that health and safety is effective, management will need to encourage all staff to be involved and committed; this is about establishing and developing a 'health and safety culture'. Health and safety culture is about positive attitudes and behaviours towards health and safety through risk reduction and accident prevention. This is achieved by adopting four key elements known as the four Cs – Control, Competence, Cooperation and Communication.

Control

Control is about ensuring that you have the systems, methods and resources in place to control risks and demonstrate safe working practice; this involves the following:

- Leading by example – developing management-led policies and procedures that demonstrate a personal commitment to health and safety
- Providing clear direction – communicating the importance of health and safety so that there is no misunderstanding about organisational standards
- Ensuring that all employees know and understand their responsibilities and how they will be held accountable
- Identifying specific responsibilities, especially where 'specialist' expertise is called for and ensuring effective delegation
- Ensuring that all persons understand their responsibilities and know how to discharge them effectively

Competence

All employees must be competent to carry out tasks safely; this involves the following:

- Assessing the capabilities at recruitment and selection

- Assessing the skills needed to carry out all activities safely
- Ensuring that the assigned competent person has the required level of knowledge and skills to perform his/her duty
- Providing the means to ensure that all employees, including temporary staff, are adequately instructed and trained
- Ensuring that people involved in significant hazardous tasks have the necessary training, skills, experience and other qualities to carry out the job safely
- Having appropriate channels in place for access to specialist advice when required

Co-operation

Developing cooperation between individuals and teams is vital to the management of health and safety. This cannot be gained by just telling people what they must do; this involves the following:

- Consulting with staff or the elected health and safety representative
- Involving people in planning, implementing, reviewing and developing procedures and solving problems.
- Involving all staff in risk assessments and the selection of suitable control measures
- Encouraging a team approach to improving safety standards, objectives and performance

It is vital to the dental practice that staff are encouraged to cooperate in developing a positive health and safety culture.

Communication

Maintaining effective communication is an important aspect in developing a health and safety culture. It is essential that the communication system is a two-way process that allows for responses from the receivers of information. Communication involves the following:

- Providing information about hazards, arrangements for risk controls and preventive measures

■ Including health and safety issues in team meetings regularly
■ Encouraging two-way communication and discussions
■ Showing others that you are taking on board their ideas

Communication is not just about sending messages, it is about making sure messages have been received in the way you intended, understood, remembered and acted upon.

3. Planning and implementing

Effective planning should be an integral part of health and safety management. The plan should be established at management level, cover all activities and clearly reflect the needs of the practice. Plans will specify how safe working practices are to be undertaken across the business. This will be stated in the form of health and safety performance standards and will set out what the practice wants to achieve. The performance standards that should be considered in dental practices are as follows:

■ All job descriptions and terms and conditions of employment contain health and safety requirements and responsibilities.
■ Health and safety behaviour is monitored and included in staff performance reviews (appraisals).
■ Safety inspections are planned and carried out routinely.
■ Risk assessments are planned, undertaken and reviewed.
■ Safe systems and operating procedures exist for all at-risk situations.
■ Emergency plans are in place.
■ Consultation and communication process with staff is in place.
■ Information, instruction, supervision and training is identified, provided and evaluated.
■ Arrangements are in place to handle accidents/significant events.
■ Audits are planned, undertaken and results acted upon.

■ The health and safety policy reflects the needs of the organisation and is reviewed periodically.
■ Health and safety records are identified, traceable and logged (Figure 12.2).

The above performance standards is not an exhaustive list but will provide direction in terms of setting health and safety performance standards which must be achieved by the organisation.

When devising performance standards the intended outcome must be clear to everyone and provide detail regarding how and when the standard must be achieved. Performance standards expressed as **S.M.A.R.T.E.R** objectives are useful in making it explicit.

■ **Specific** – the standard defines precisely what must be achieved and by whom.
■ **Measurable** – it states how performance will be assessed against the set standard.
■ **Achievable** – a realistic and reasonable amount of effort and application has been considered so the standard can be achieved.
■ **Realistic** – standards are practical and the necessary resources are available. A realistic health and safety standard is usually set by legislation; the term 'reasonably practicable' is often used.
■ **Time based** – a set time should be specified when you want to achieve or carry out the standard. This enables outcomes to be assessed within a given period.
■ **Ethical** – performance standards must be in line with legal and professional requirements; they must demonstrate equality of opportunity and a duty of care to all persons.
■ **Recorded** – standards should be recorded to demonstrate commitment, facilitate communication, develop understanding and assist with review.

All staff should be involved in the setting of objectives to ensure that a team commitment is demonstrated in achieving targets; it is important that all persons are clear as to their level of involvement. Health and safety performance

Figure 12.2   Health and safety document log.

Record/document title	Location	Issue no. and date	Review date

Health and safety documents must be identifiable, traceable and maintained on the above log. Retention periods must be established in-line with legal and professional requirements.

standards are implemented to assist in managing risks which are present within the day-to-day operations of the practice; standards help to demonstrate that risk control is effective.

4. Monitor and measure performance

As with all other business activities you need to measure the health and safety performance against the agreed standard to find out if you are being successful and achieving your objectives. You need to know

- where you are at the moment;
- where you want to be;
- what is the difference and why?

Performance measurement is an ongoing and frequent process and should be carried out by the manager or immediate supervisor. The frequency will need to be determined by the practice; in some instances, it may be stated in law, for example, 'the periodic examination of autoclaves must be at least every 14 months'. Performance is monitored by using two specific methods – active and reactive monitoring. Both play a vital part in assessing if objectives have been met and if not, why not.

Active monitoring

This is also termed 'proactive monitoring' and is designed to measure the achievement of objectives and standards before incidents occur. It involves regular checks and inspections to ensure standards are being met, management controls are effectively implemented and the required actions are taken to remedy defects.

Reactive monitoring

This system is used to collect and analyse information after things have gone wrong. It involves an examination of records relating to accident statistics and investigation, significant event analysis, cases of ill health, sickness absence, property or equipment damage and near misses to help determine why performance was not to the standard set.

The following are all examples of monitoring systems:

- **Safety inspections** – Generally, a safety inspection is an examination of premises or a specific area in the organisation. The purpose is to check if premises are being maintained and, therefore, duties are being carried out in accordance with set standards and procedures. Inspections should have a clear specification, that is, a check list, be planned and carried out at regular intervals and made known to the rest of the team.
- **Observation of working practices and on-the-job discussions** – This is best carried out by monitoring the performance of an individual against the safe operating procedure. It requires an understanding of the procedure and knowledge of the subject in order to determine if the individual is carrying out safe working practices. It can be supplemented by questioning and discussion provided this does not disrupt the activity or render it unsafe.
- **Task analysis** – This system can eliminate the hazards or control the risks of a particular activity; the analysis isolates each single task, examines the individual hazards and indicates remedies to control risks. It involves the critical examination of equipment and processes, systems of work, influences on behaviour, the qualification and training required for the job and the degree of instruction, supervision and control which is necessary.
- **Safety walk tours** – This is a visual examination of a work area and can be carried out by any member of the team or other persons. It is usually an unplanned observation of all aspects of the working environment. For safety tours to be effective, it is essential that any deficiencies identified during the tour are remedied immediately and communicated to all concerned.
- **Health and safety surveys** – These are detailed examinations of a number of critical areas of operation or an in-depth study of the whole health and safety operation of premises. A survey might examine in great detail any aspect of health and safety. A survey report is

then published; in most cases, this report is purely critical and produced on an observation and recommendation basis. A survey report is mainly concerned with risks and the system for bringing about a gradual upgrading of standards. The aim of the report is to plan a phased programme of health and safety improvement over a period of time.

- **Environmental monitoring** – This type of system is generally associated with hazardous substances and ionising radiation. It is a complex technique that produces both qualitative and quantitative results and can be used to measure personal and environmental doses.

Information from active and reactive monitoring should be used to identify situations that create risks and implement procedures to eliminate or adequately control the risks. Priority should be given to where risks are greatest and where the potential of serious harm exists. You will need to determine the most suitable monitoring system for your dental practice to meet the needs of the organisation.

5. Performance review and audit

Monitoring provides the information to enable you to review activities and decide how to improve performance. Review and auditing is a planned process and consists of the following:

Performance review

The performance review process helps to make a judgement on whether the performance standards are being met and if the Health and Safety Policy is being implemented and if the objectives are being achieved. Policy review is best planned and scheduled over a given period, that is, 12 months (Figures 12.3 and 12.4). This ensures that it is an ongoing and consistent process and will assist in prioritising areas for concern which were identified during the monitoring stage. It will help to identify what needs to be done in order to rectify and thereby improve performance.

Audit

Health and safety auditing enables the practice to determine whether the management planning and control system is valid and reliable (Figure 12.5). The two main objectives of an audit are as follows:

- To ensure that the standards achieved meet the objectives set out in the safety policy
- To provide information to justify continuation of the same strategy or determine areas which need to change, that is, act on the audit results

It must be clear that an audit is not the same as an inspection; the audit is a systematic assessment/examination of the organisation's safety management system and procedures. This includes policy development, organising the

Figure 12.3   Health and safety policy review.

AUDIT PERIOD:		DATE AUDIT COMPLETED:			
1. Policy					
Standard	**Yes**	**No**	**N/A**	**Comments and date**	
1.1 Roles and responsibilities clearly defined?					
1.2 Policy brought to the attention of all relevant persons?					
1.3 Policy reviewed since last audit?					
1.4 Policy revisions consulted on before implementation?					
1.5 Employees informed of revisions to the policy?					
1.6 Policy appropriate to the organisation?					

Figure 12.3   (*continued*)

Standard	Yes	No	N/A	Comments and date
2. Accidents and first aid				
2.1 Staff aware of the need to report all accidents including significant events?				
2.2 Accident report forms available?				
2.3 Staff aware of requirements and responsibilities under RIDDOR?				
2.4 Accident investigation and significant event analysis undertaken, reports completed and data protected?				
2.5 Corrective action taken and controls implemented to prevent recurrence?				
2.6 First aid kit available and fully stocked?				
2.7 Staff aware of first aid kit location?				
2.8 Relevant staff received first aid training?				
3. Alcohol, drugs and smoking				
3.1 Alcohol or drug misuse identified?				
3.2 Assistance provided to help with problem?				
3.3 Alcohol or drug misuse issues dealt with through disciplinary action (staff only)?				
3.4 Smoke-free workplace rule communicated?				
3.5 Disregard for smoke-free rule identified and dealt with through disciplinary action (staff only)?				
3.6 Drug, alcohol and smoking issues resolved through above means?				
4. Communication and training				
4.1 Induction undertaken and recorded for all new staff?				
4.2 Staff trained to statutory and in-house standards?				
4.3 Ongoing training needs identified and provided for all staff?				
4.4 Provision of training evaluated to assess effectiveness?				
4.5 Training records held for all staff?				
4.6 Staff meetings held routinely and minutes taken?				
4.7 Staff meetings enable opinions, views and feedback from all persons?				
4.8 Outcomes of meetings are acted upon?				
5. Conflict management				
5.1 Conflict management risk assessments undertaken?				
5.2 Risks evaluated and preventive measures implemented?				

(*continued overleaf*)

Figure 12.3   *(continued)*

Standard	Yes	No	N/A	Comments and date
5.3 Actual situations of conflict happened?				
5.4 Situations investigated and analysed for root causes?				
5.5 Situations managed effectively and amicably resolved?				
5.6 Situations recorded?				
5.7 Conflict management training provided?				
6. Disability access				
6.1 Disabled access assessment undertaken?				
6.2 Areas for improvement identified?				
6.3 Access improvements implemented?				
6.4 Disability awareness training provided?				
7. Display screen equipment				
7.1 DSE assessments undertaken and recorded?				
7.2 Improvements made to workstations as a result of the assessment?				
7.3 Staff informed and trained on safe use of DSE?				
7.4 Staff applies safe working practices when using DSE?				
7.5 Staff provided with eye sight tests on their request? (where applicable)				
8. Electrical safety				
8.1 Mains electrical circuits adequate for requirements?				
8.2 Arrangements in place for inspection of both fixed and portable systems?				
8.3 Electricity maintenance programme in place?				
8.4 Use of competent persons enlisted to carry out above procedures?				
8.5 Emergencies/disasters identified and rectified?				
9. Fire safety and emergency				
9.1 Fire and emergency risk assessments undertaken?				
9.2 Competent person appointed to manage fire safety/emergencies?				
9.3 Means of access and egress satisfactory?				
9.4 Fire-fighting appliances provided and maintained?				
9.5 Staff trained in fire-fighting and evacuation procedures?				
9.6 Fire drills undertaken and recorded?				
9.7 Outcomes of fire drills acted upon?				

Figure 12.3   (*continued*)

Standard	Yes	No	N/A	Comments and date
10. Hazardous substances				
10.1 Hazardous substances identified?				
10.2 COSHH assessments undertaken?				
10.3 Control measures implemented and followed?				
10.4 Assessments communicated and staff trained?				
11. Infection control				
11.1 Up to date legislation and professional standards sourced and communicated?				
11.2 Development plans in place to meet up to date requirements?				
11.3 Staff trained on standards required?				
11.4 Immunisation records held for all relevant staff?				
11.5 Occupational health service introduced and communicated?				
11.6 All documents and records completed and retained?				
12. Lone working				
12.1 Lone workers identified?				
12.2 Assessments undertaken?				
12.3 Controls implemented?				
12.4 Assessments and controls communicated to relevant people?				
13. Management systems				
13.1 There is a line of control and authority for health and safety?				
13.2 Staff are made aware of their roles and responsibilities for health and safety?				
13.3 Organisational health and safety objectives are set and communicated?				
13.4 Staff set their own objectives for health and safety?				
13.5 Routine inspections undertaken by all staff?				
13.6 Results of inspections acted upon and corrective action taken where necessary?				
13.7 Random sample audits undertaken and one to one interviews, findings and results acted upon?				
13.8 Commitment to continuous improvement is actively demonstrated?				
14. Manual handling				
14.1 Manual handling activities with the potential to harm are avoided?				

(*continued overleaf*)

Figure 12.3   (*continued*)

Standard	Yes	No	N/A	Comments and date
14.2 Manual handling assessments undertaken to include: load, individual, task and environment?				
14.3 Preventive and protective measures implemented?				
14.4 Staff have been trained?				
15. Medical emergencies				
15.1 Staff training received?				
15.2 Training is recorded?				
15.3 Staff aware of procedures in event of medical emergencies?				
15.4 Medical emergencies dealt with effectively?				
15.5 Medical emergencies recorded?				
15.6 Emergency drugs sourced and stock controlled by competent person?				
16. Occupational health and well-being				
16.1 Assessments undertaken to identify at risk factors?				
16.2 Preventive measures implemented?				
16.3 Medical screening to identify individual needs?				
16.4 Results of screening acted upon to minimise risk to health and well-being?				
16.5 Health promotion programmes provided to staff?				
16.6 Return to work support for those who are absent for period of time?				
16.7 Use of external sources to assist, that is, occupational health service?				
17. Personal protective equipment				
17.1 Appropriate PPE made available?				
17.2 Staff trained on the use of PPE and training recorded?				
17.3 PPE used and worn when necessary?				
17.4 PPE removed before entering into non-clinical areas?				
17.5 PPE not worn outside of the practice?				
17.6 PPE maintained?				
17.7 PPE defects reported and acted upon?				
18. Radiation protection				
18.1 HSE notified of use of X-ray equipment?				
18.2 Controlled area identified and local rules displayed?				
18.3 Risk assessment undertaken?				

Figure 12.3 (*continued*)

Standard	Yes	No	N/A	Comments and date
18.4 RPA and RPS appointed?				
18.5 Ionising radiation operators received training?				
18.6 Training recorded?				
18.7 Directing the exposure restricted to trained and qualified staff and a record held?				
18.8 Inventory of equipment maintained?				
18.9 Dose meter monitoring provided where applicable?				
18.10 All procedures comply with the quality assurance programme?				
19. Risk assessment				
19.1 Significant hazards identified?				
19.2 Risks have been evaluated?				
19.3 Control measures implemented?				
19.4 Risk assessments recorded (five or more employees)?				
19.5 Staff involved, consulted and informed?				
19.6 Training needs identified as a result of risk assessments?				
19.7 Risk assessments reviewed and revised if necessary?				
20. Stress management				
20.1 Significant causes of stress identified?				
20.2 Range of methods used to analyse causes and contributory factors?				
20.3 Promote active discussion to decide practical improvements?				
20.4 Implement preventive measures?				
20.5 Monitor working patterns to assess stress factors?				
20.6 Provide support for those who report concerns or are absent?				
21. Visitors, locums and contractors				
21.1 Sign in and out procedure implemented at all times?				
21.2 Information and instruction provided and understanding confirmed?				
21.3 Relevant policy items communicated?				
21.4 Rules complied with at all times?				
21.5 Problems identified and acted upon?				
21.6 Non-conformances recorded?				

(*continued overleaf*)

Figure 12.3   (*continued*)

Standard	Yes	No	N/A	Comments and date
22. Work equipment				
22.1 Safe operating procedures for all necessary equipment?				
22.2 Safe operating procedures displayed and/or accessible?				
22.3 Safe operating procedures communicated and training provided?				
22.4 Staff adheres to safe operating procedures?				
22.5 Visual equipment checks undertaken and recorded?				
22.6 Maintenance procedures arranged and undertaken?				
22.7 Maintenance records completed and held?				
22.8 Defects and rectifications identified and corrected immediately?				
23. Working environment and welfare facilities				
23.1 Housekeeping and general cleaning is undertaken to an acceptable standard?				
23.2 Workplace maintained in good repair?				
23.3 Heating, lighting, ventilation and temperature of acceptable standard?				
23.4 Floors and traffic routes free from obstructions?				
23.5 Staircases secure and handrail provided?				
23.6 Adequate supply of drinking water supplied?				
23.7 Toilet and washing facilities provided and maintained?				
23.8 Facilities for rest and eating meals are away from any risk of contamination?				
24. Working hours				
24.1 Staff including young persons informed of legal limits?				
24.2 Staff informed of daily, weekly and in-work rest breaks?				
24.3 Hours of work analysed and monitored?				
24.4 Additional employment staff may have established?				
24.5 Corrective action taken where excessive hours identified?				
24.6 Hours of work altered for disabled staff where necessary?				
DATE AUDIT COMPLETED				
PERSON SIGNING OFF AUDIT				
AUDIT REPORT DATED				

Figure 12.4 Health and safety policy review schedule.

AUDIT PERIOD: (Insert year start and end)

MONTH (Insert month in each shaded box)

Policy Arrangement												
1. Accidents and first aid												
2. Alcohol, drugs and smoking												
3. Communication and training												
4. Conflict management												
5. Disabled access												
6. Display screen equipment												
7. Electrical safety												
8. Fire/emergency procedures												
9. Hazardous substances												
10. Infection control												
11. Lone working												
12. Management systems												
13. Manual handling												
14. Medical emergencies												
15. Occupational health and WB												
16. PPE												
17. Radiation protection												
18. Risk assessment												
19. Stress management												
20. Visitors, locums, contractors												
21. Work equipment												
22. Working environment												
23. Working hours												

All policy arrangements must be reviewed within the 12-month period.

Indicate when each policy arrangement will be reviewed by shading the relevant month (see the above example for arrangements 1 and 2).

It is envisaged that two policy items will be reviewed each month.

team, planning and implementation, monitoring and measuring performance and performance review and audit. If the template provided (Figure 12.5) is designed to be used for an initial audit if you have not carried out this process before, it can then be adapted for subsequent audits to meet the individual needs of the practice. Following the audit, an audit report should be compiled, clearly stating the results and the required action; this should be discussed with and issued to the employer and the findings circulated to all members of the team (Figure 12.6).

The general principles of health and safety management will apply to all dental practices, regardless of the size. However, you may want to tailor them to meet your specific needs.

Summary

A well thought out health and safety management process helps the organisation to prevent accidents and ill health. It demonstrates a tangible commitment to employees and anyone else who

Figure 12.5   Management systems audit.

PERSON CONDUCTING AUDIT:		AUDIT DATE:		
1. Policy				
Standard	**Yes**	**No**	**Comment**	
1.1 Is the policy appropriate to the nature and scale of the organisation's health and safety risks?				
1.2 Does it include a commitment to continual improvement?				
1.3 Does it include a commitment to at least comply with current applicable health and safety legislation and other professional requirements?				
1.4 Is it documented, implemented and maintained?				
1.5 Is it communicated to all employees with the intent that they are made aware of their individual organisation's health and safety responsibilities?				
1.6 Is it made available to interested parties?				
1.7 Is it reviewed periodically to ensure that it remains relevant and appropriate to the organisation?				
2. Organise the team				
Standard	**Yes**	**No**	**Comments**	
2.1 Are the roles, responsibilities and authority for those who 'manage', perform or verify activities, which have an effect on the health and safety risks, documented and communicated?				
2.2 Has the organisation appointed someone from 'management' to take ultimate responsibility for health and safety to ensure systems are properly implemented and performing to the requirements?				
2.3 Does the organisation have procedures to ensure personnel are competent to perform tasks that may impact on health and safety?				

Figure 12.5   (*continued*)

Standard	Yes	No	Comment
2.4 Does the organisation have procedures to ensure staff are aware of the importance of and conformance to health and safety policy and procedures?			
2.5 Does the organisation have procedures to ensure staff are aware of the consequences of their work activities and the benefits of improved personal performance?			
2.6 Does the organisation have procedures to ensure staff are aware of their roles and responsibilities in achieving conformance to health and safety policy and emergency preparations and response requirements?			
2.7 Does the organisation have procedures for ensuring that health and safety information is communicated to and from employees and other interested parties?			
2.8 Are communication and consultation arrangements documented?			
2.9 Are employees involved in the development and review of policies and procedures in order to manage risks?			
2.10 Are employees consulted where there are changes that affect health and safety?			
2.11 Are staff represented on organisation's health and safety matters?			
2.12 Has management provided suitable and sufficient resources for the implementation, control and improvement of health and safety management system?			
2.13 Does management produce and control reports/records on the performance of the health and safety management system and communicate them to staff?			

3. Planning and implementation			
Standard	**Yes**	**No**	**Comments**
3.1 Are procedures in place for the ongoing identification of hazards, assessment of risks and the implementation of controls?			
3.2 Does 3.1 include routine and non-routine activities?			
3.3 Does 3.1 include the activities of all personnel having access to the workplace (including contractors, locums and visitors)?			
3.4 Does 3.1 include facilities at the premises?			
3.5 Is the methodology for identifying hazards and assessing risks clearly defined, planned and timed to ensure it is proactive?			
3.6 Does the RA process enable risks to be classified and eliminated or controlled using the hierarchy of controls?			
3.7 Does the RA process enable training needs to be identified?			

(*continued overleaf*)

Figure 12.5   (*continued*)

Standard	Yes	No	Comment
3.8 Does the RA process include monitoring of required actions to ensure the effectiveness and timeliness of their implementation?			
3.9 Does the RA process include at least an annual review of all RAs and revision where necessary?			
3.10 Does the organisation have a procedure for identifying and accessing legal and professional health and safety applicable requirements?			
3.11 Are the RAs kept up to date and communicated to relevant and interested parties?			
3.12 Does the organisation establish health and safety objectives for each function, that is, clinical, non-clinical etc.?			
3.13 Are the objectives in 3.12 reviewed to ensure they are **S.M.A.R.T.E.R**; are all interested parties involved in the review and do they demonstrate continual improvement?			
3.14 Is the organisation's health and safety management programme reviewed at regular intervals and revised accordingly?			
3.15 Does the organisation have documented SOPs for all at-risk operations/activities and are these accessible and communicated?			
3.16 Does the organisation establish and maintain plans to identify the potential for and response to incidents and emergency situations, for example, power failure/cut, fire, water leak, flood, burglary, medical emergency and physical attack?			
3.17 Are the above plans aimed at preventing and mitigating illness and injury and are the plans reviewed periodically?			
3.18 Are the above procedures tested periodically and outcomes acted upon, for example, fire drill, use of backup generator, simulated physical attack and CPD?			
4. Monitor and measure performance			
Standard	Yes	No	Comments
4.1 Does the organisation monitor and measure if health and safety objectives are met?			
4.2 Does the organisation use proactive measures of performance to monitor compliance with criteria, legislation and professional standards?			
4.3 Does the organisation use reactive measures of performance, that is, monitor accidents, ill health, incidents and near misses?			
4.4 Does the organisation record data and results of monitoring and measurement to facilitate corrective and preventative action analysis?			

Figure 12.5 (*continued*)

Standard	Yes	No	Comment
4.5 Does the organisation establish and define responsibility and authority for the handling and investigation of accidents, incidents, non-conformances?			
4.6 Does the organisation take action to mitigate consequences arising from accidents, incidents or non-conformances (i.e. through risk assessment)?			
4.7 Does the organisation initiate and complete corrective and preventive actions (i.e. through risk assessment)?			
4.8 Does the organisation confirm the effectiveness of corrective and preventive actions?			
4.9 Are health and safety records identifiable and traceable to the activities involved?			
4.10 Is the health and safety audit programme established and maintained?			
4.11 Does the health and safety audit programme review the results of previous audits?			
4.12 Does the health and safety audit programme provide valid, reliable and sufficient results of audits?			

5. Performance review and audit

Standard	Yes	No	Comments
5.1 Does top management review health and safety systems to ensure suitability, adequacy and effectiveness?			
5.2 Does the management review process ensure that the necessary information is collected to allow an evaluation?			
5.3 Does the management review address the possible need for changes to policy, objectives and any other elements of health and safety in the light of audit results, changing circumstances and the commitment to continual improvement?			
5.4 Is the management review process documented?			

Additional comments:

Signatures are required to confirm agreement to the above audit process

Manager's signature and name	**Employer's signature and name**

Figure 12.6 Management systems audit report.

REPORT PERIOD:	
REPORT DATED:	
REPORT COMPILED BY:	
POSITION IN ORGANISATION:	
REPORT CIRCULATED TO THE PEOPLE NAMED BELOW:	
DATE CIRCULATED:	METHOD:
Name	**Position**

This report is based on the findings of the management review undertaken over the last 12-month period as stated above.

1. Audit process and objectives
2. Exclusions (items not reviewed) and reasons

Figure 12.6 (*continued*)

3. Good practice identified (compliance with policy)
4. Non-conformances
5. Action required (by whom and when)
6. Opportunities for improvement (agree on reasonable plan)

may be affected. It helps to integrate health and safety with all other management functions and gives confidence to staff and patients alike that their health, safety, welfare and well-being are at the forefront of the organisation's operations.

Action – check the following

- Have you assessed where you are at now and the current health and safety status of your business?
- Can you actively and consciously demonstrate how you manage health and safety?

- Do you need to do anything else to improve the management of health and safety?
- Have you identified if your business is at risk as a result of health and safety?

Frequently asked questions

Q. How do we develop a safety culture?

A. A safety culture takes time to develop throughout the practice as it requires the positive involvement and commitment from all staff. Staff will need to be encouraged and motivated in order to recognise the tangible benefits to them and to the organisation. Management should ensure that people possess the necessary skills and knowledge to carry out their duties safely, provide direction and guidance, facilitate a two-way communication process and organise work activities to enable objectives to be met.

Q. How often should we carry out a health and safety audit?

A. Auditing enables management to ensure that their policy is being carried out and that the health and safety management system is achieving the desired outcomes. The timing of an audit should reflect the needs of the organisation and be conducted according to the health and safety plan as indicated in the performance standards. However, it is good practice to audit your systems and procedures annually.

Links to other chapters

Although all of the chapters within this manual have general reference to 'Managing Health and Safety' the following chapters are of specific reference:

Chapter 3 – Communication and training
Chapter 17 – Policy
Chapter 19 – Risk assessment

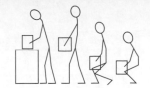

13 Manual handling

Scope of this chapter

- Introduction
- Legislation
- Manual handling injuries
- Manual handling: Stage 1 – avoid tasks
- Manual handling: Stage 2 – assess risks
- Manual handling: Stage 3 – reduce injury
- Training

Figures

Figure 13.1 – Manual handling activities assessment.
Figure 13.2 – Manual handling risk assessment.

Introduction

Manual handling activities can cause many types of injury and most commonly affect the back and upper limbs. Almost one-third of injuries reported to the enforcing authority have been attributed to the manual handling of loads. All dental environments carry out some form of manual handling operations which involve an individual moving or supporting objects. This may include lifting the object and putting it down, or pushing or pulling the load. In dentistry, we must consider the nature of the load as it could be an inanimate object or a person. These activities must be assessed in order to identify how the activity may cause injury and determine appropriate steps to reduce the risk of injury to the lowest level possible.

Legislation

- Health and Safety at Work etc. Act 1974:

  Employers have a general duty to their employees, so far as is reasonable, to ensure safety and absence of risk to health in the use, handling, storage and transport of articles and substances.

- Manual Handling Operations Regulations 1992:

  Employers are required to avoid manual handling activities where there is a foreseeable risk of injury, if it is not possible to avoid the activity, than a risk assessment should be undertaken to reduce the risk of injury.

- Management of Health and Safety at Work Regulations 1999:

  Employers must undertake suitable and sufficient assessments of risks to the health and safety of employees and implement reasonable controls.

Manual handling injuries

The injuries and health problems that may result from incorrect handling techniques and poor systems of work are numerous. The most common types of manual handling injuries are as follows:

- Cuts and bruises to the fingers, hands and feet
- Sprained ligaments
- Sprained and inflamed tendons
- Trapped nerves
- Ruptured and displaced discs
- Hernias
- Fractures
- Stress fractures

To add to the problem, injuries may not occur as a result of a single event and might therefore not be recognised immediately. Repeated exposure to the activity over time may result in more long-term effects and, in severe cases, disability. In addition to the injuries sustained by the person carrying out the activity, we must also consider others in the immediate vicinity who may be at risk from the activity. In particular, if the task involves moving a person they may also be injured if this is carried out incorrectly.

Manual handling: Stage 1 – avoid tasks

Avoidance of the manual handling activities, which present a **foreseeable** risk and therefore could result in injury, must be the first consideration in all instances. In order to determine if a risk exists, you first need to identify the type of activities that constitute 'manual handling'.

Identify manual handling activities

This can be done by observing people carrying out their day-to-day duties, talking to staff to establish if they have any concerns or individual needs and referring to significant event analysis and accident reports (Figure 13.1). To assist in identifying activities, it is useful to break them down into tasks as follows:

- Lifting
- Carrying
- Pushing
- Pulling

The information gathered will help to determine if activities present a foreseeable risk which needs to be addressed. It may be that all manual handling activities are identified as presenting a risk. However, in some instances the risk may be negligible. For example, in the transportation of one instrument tray from the surgery to the decontamination area, the manual handling risk is negligible while the risk of transmitting infection is greater. Table 13.1 will help to determine if a foreseeable risk is present from **lifting and lowering** a load. This table provides **guideline weights** for men and women who, when lifting in that zone, would normally be safe. It is not an authoritative account of the weight everyone can handle as other factors will need to be considered.

Care must be taken not to overlook any aspects and if there is any doubt about the level of risk, then steps must be taken to either avoid or reduce it to as low as is possible. The next step is to decide if the task can be avoided. This is done by the following:

- Elimination – remove the need to move the load, for example, by asking suppliers for smaller packages of items or moving the stock room closer to where the load is delivered.
- Mechanising – provide a trolley to move items of stock.

Where avoidance is not possible an overall risk rating should be assigned to the activity and then the next step is to carry out a manual handling assessment.

Figure 13.1   Manual handling activities assessment.

NO:	DATE:		NAME OF ASSESSOR:
INITIAL ASSESSMENT (✓)		REASSESSMENT (✓)	LOCATION:

1. Brief description of activity being assessed

2. Tasks involved in activity (brief description)	
Lifting	Carrying
Pushing	Pulling
3. Persons carrying out the activity (names and job titles)	4. Individual needs/vulnerable persons
5. Activity presents a foreseeable risk? Yes/No (if yes go to 6; if no go to 10.)	6. Activity can be avoided Yes/No (if yes go to 7; if no go to 8.)
7. Avoided (specify); then go to 10 Eliminated: Mechanised:	8. Overall assessment of risk (risk rating) Low/Med/High (go to 9. Full assessment required)
9. Date of full assessment using Stage 2:	10. Date to review activity (specify)
Assessor's position:	Assessor's signature:

Table 13.1 Guideline weights for men and women.

Zone	Load held close to body	Load held at arm's length
Full height (arms above head)	Men – 10 kg Women – 5 kg	Men – 5 kg Women – 3.5 kg
Shoulder height	Men – 20 kg Women – 10 kg	Men – 10 kg Women – 5 kg
Elbow height	Men – 25 kg Women – 12.5 kg	Men – 15 kg Women – 7.5 kg
Knuckle height	Men – 20 kg Women – 10 kg	Men – 10 kg Women – 5 kg
Mid-lower leg height	Men – 10 kg Women – 5 kg	Men – 5 kg Women – 3.5 kg

Manual handling: Stage 2 – assess risks

Where the assessment of activities shows that the risk cannot be avoided, a full risk assessment must be undertaken to identify how people may be harmed or injured. The information gathered in Stage 1 and the overall risk rating will help to prioritise the assessment. When carrying out Stage 2, it is important to once again involve the people who are undertaking the activities in order to obtain accurate and reliable information based on 'real life' events as they actually happen. This involves an ergonomic approach to assessing manual handling activities (Figure 13.2), which considers the following four factors:

- Load – weight, shape, height etc.
- Individual capability – personal factors or needs of person/s undertaking the activity.
- Task – what does it involve, for example, repetitive movement or reaching etc.?
- Environment – are there any limitations on movement or are there slippery surfaces etc.?

The above-mentioned approach is often termed the *L.I.T.E assessment* of manual handling activities. Each aspect of the above factors should be assessed and a risk rating assigned. If remedial action is required this must be stated in order of priority and a summary of the assessment completed, indicting an overall risk rating.

Manual handling: Stage 3 – reduce injury

Having completed the assessment in Stage 2, the manual handling activity must now be further analysed and appropriate steps taken to reduce the risk of injury to the lowest level reasonably practicable. The overall risk rating will determine the action priority and this must once again involve the persons who have been identified as being involved in the activity and therefore at risk. When taking remedial action the same factors used to assess the risk should be referred to and corrective action determined.

Load

- Compact the items by making them smaller and more manageable.
- Lighten the load by splitting it into smaller packages.
- Ask suppliers to deliver in smaller quantities.
- Grasp the load by using handles or grips.
- Check packages for sharp edges or wear personal protective equipment (PPE) if necessary.
- Secure the contents to avoid them moving around.
- If the activity involves moving a person, effective communication is vital. The person should be asked if he/she needs assistance. He/she may prefer to be independent or may be accompanied by a carer.

Individual capability

- Never allow the movement of objects that are too heavy or beyond a person's physical capabilities.
- Ensure that health problems or physical conditions are communicated.
- Consider the needs of vulnerable groups, for example, women of child-bearing age, young

persons and those with pre-existing conditions. Pre-employment medical screening should be carried out.

- Be aware of certain conditions, for example, pregnancy, where the unborn child must also be considered.
- Provide training on moving and handling techniques.
- Encourage those who are unsure about the activity to seek advice and assistance.

Task

- Encourage people to hold the load closer to the body.
- Ensure that the body is being used efficiently, for example, using strong leg muscles.
- Consider team handling of loads.
- Avoid moving loads over long distances.
- Store loads at waist height where possible.
- Split the lift movement into two motions. For example, use a two-stage lift technique.
- Avoid repetition of movement.
- Reduce the frequency of the activity.

Environment

- Assess the area before moving loads.
- Remove any obstacles which infringe on the space around the lifting activity.
- Clean up spillages before proceeding and ensure good housekeeping.
- Ensure that lighting is adequate and suitable for the activity.
- Ensure that the area is well ventilated and has a suitable temperature.
- Avoid the need to go up or downstairs while moving the load.
- Where possible, store loads on the same level as they arrive into the practice.

Risk assessment must have a planned monitoring date to ensure that the controls are effective in controlling risks and a planned review date to ensure that it remains accurate, current and valid. Where five or more people are employed the Management of Health and Safety at Work Regulations require employers to record the significant findings.

Training

Where manual handling activities are routinely carried out a level of training will usually be required. It is important that training meets the needs of the practice and is tailored to the activities being undertaken and is, therefore, fit for the purpose. Most training programmes should include the following:

- How potentially hazardous loads can be recognised
- How to deal with unfamiliar loads
- When and how to use handling aids correctly
- When and how to use personal protective equipment
- Features of the working environment that contribute to safety
- The importance of good housekeeping
- Correct handling techniques. Basic techniques are as follows:
  - ☐ Plan and prepare the activity, consider what is being moved, and check the weight of the load.
  - ☐ The body should be positioned with feet slightly apart, distributing the weight evenly.
  - ☐ Lift by bending the knees, keeping the back straight, get a firm grip around the base of the load and lift in stages.
  - ☐ Move the load, keeping it close to the body and ensuring that the view ahead is unrestricted.
  - ☐ Lower the load by reversing the lift movement. Avoid putting the load down on fingers or toes and ensure that it is secure in its final position.

Manual handling training should start at induction and should not be a one-off. It must be reviewed periodically to reinforce the importance of safety. Work activities should be monitored to ensure that people are applying safe manual handling techniques. Records of training should be maintained to demonstrate commitment to continuing professional development.

Figure 13.2   Manual handling risk assessment.

REF TO STAGE 1 NO:	DATE:		NAME OF ASSESSOR:
LOCATION:		**IF ACTION IS REQUIRED SEE PAGE 2**	

Hazard rate (HR)	Risk rate (RR)	Action priority (AP)
A Death, major injury, major damage **B** Over 3-day injury; damage to property/equipment **C** Minor injury, minor damage to property	**1.** Extremely likely to occur **2.** Frequent/often/likely to occur **3.** Slight chance of occurring	**A1 –** Unacceptable; must receive immediate attention before work continues **A2/B1 –** Urgent; must receive attention as soon as possible to remove hazard or reduce risk **A3/C1 –** Must receive attention to reduce risk **B2 –** Should receive attention to reduce risk **B3/C2 –** Low priority; reduce risk after other priorities **C3 –** Very low priority; reduce hazard or risk after other priorities

Risk factor	No	Yes	HR	RR	AP	Action Y/N
The load – is it?						
Bulky or of an odd shape						
Heavier than the guidelines						
Difficult to hold or grasp						
Harmful – hot, sharp or otherwise						
Unstable/unpredictable in movement						
The individual capability – does the job?						
Require unusual strength or height						
Pose a risk due to an existing health problem						
Pose a risk due to pregnancy						
Require additional information/training						
Require you to be supervised						
The task – does it involve?						
Holding loads away from the trunk						
Twisting						
Stooping						
Reaching above shoulder height						
Carrying over long distances						
Strenuous pushing or pulling						
Repetitive handling						
Frequent handling (every day)						
Regular handling (every week)						

Figure 13.2 *(continued)*

Risk factor	No	Yes	HR	RR	AP	Action Y/N
The environment – are there?						
Confined spaces which limit movement						
Uneven and unstable floors						
Slippery surface						
Poor lighting conditions						
Hot, cold and humid conditions						
Steps and stairs to encounter						

Action in order of priority to control the activity	Date to be completed by	Date completed
1.		
2.		
3.		
4.		
5.		
6.		
7.		
8.		
9.		
10.		

Summary of assessment
Manual handling activities covered by this assessment:
Names and job titles of people who carry out this activity: (if different from Stage 1)
Any other comments:
Overall risk rating:

Date for review of assessment:	Assessor's signature:

Summary

Manual handling should be avoided wherever possible. Where it cannot be avoided, an assessment must be undertaken, risks reduced as low as possible and the activity made safer by implementing suitable and appropriate control measures. The assessment methods discussed in this chapter should be suitable and sufficient for dental settings. However, if any of the controls cannot be reasonably applied then a more detailed assessment will be required.

Action – check the following

- Have you assessed all manual handling activities?
- Have staff been informed of the manual handling activities they undertake which could put them at risk?
- Have you assessed the capabilities of staff to carry out manual handling activities safely?

Frequently asked questions

Q. Do we have to assess every manual handling activity?

A. The activities that require an assessment are those where there is a foreseeable risk of injury. You should consider all the activities where a load is moved, remembering that a load could be a person or an item. Then determine if there is a risk of injury. If the answer is 'no' you need to do no more than review the activity; if the outcome is 'yes' then a risk assessment should be undertaken.

Q. If manual handling training is provided does this have to be delivered by an expert?

A. Not necessarily; the level and nature of training will depend on the risks involved in the activities you have assessed. Training must not be used as a priority control measure or in isolation. When it comes to controlling risks, the priority should be to look at changing working practices or altering the environment before considering training.

Links to other chapters

Chapter 3 – Communication and training
Chapter 6 – Display screen equipment
Chapter 19 – Risk assessment

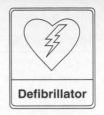

Defibrillator

14 Medical emergencies

Scope of this chapter

- Introduction
- Legislation
- Common causes and types
- Minimise the risk
- Managing medical emergencies
- Basic life support (BLS)

Figures

Figure 14.1 – Medical emergencies training log.

Introduction

In the event of a patient becoming ill in the dental surgery, the dental team must be able to act quickly to help prevent the illness or injury from becoming worse. When a patient enters the surgery the full responsibility for his/her care, which includes health, safety and welfare, is in the hands of the dentist and the team. A patient may become ill at any time while in the surgery and this could be as a result of dental treatment or because of an existing condition. It is of utmost importance that the dental team is able to recognise signs and symptoms and act quickly and effectively in a potentially life-or-death scenario.

Legislation

- Management of Health and Safety at Work Regulations 1999:

  Employers should investigate the cause of medical emergencies/accidents which is an essential part of effective health and safety management and therefore forms part of the risk assessment process. The outcome of investigations could identify the need for additional controls.

- Health and Safety at Work, etc. Act 1974:

  Employers must ensure the health, safety and welfare of employees and others who may be affected by his activities.

- Reporting of Injuries, Diseases and Dangerous Occurrences Regulations (1995) (RIDDOR):

  Requires certain incidents to be reported to the Health and Safety Executive (HSE) if they arise out of or in connection with the work being undertaken. Incidents must be reported which result in a fatality, or a member of the public being taken to hospital or suffering a major injury.

Additional requirements for RIDDOR reporting are covered in Chapter 1.

Common causes and types

Common causes

There are many reasons why a medical emergency may happen; however, the following are the most common:

- Patient anxious and nervous about the treatment and therefore feeling stressed
- Patient suffering from dental pain
- Patient suffering from physical exertion
- Patient not understanding or carrying out post-operative instructions
- Patient's existing medical condition
- Patient abuse of drugs or alcohol
- Inadequate medical history obtained
- Medical history not routinely updated
- A reaction to local anaesthetic
- The result of an accident, for example, the patient swallowing or inhaling an endodontic instrument

Common types

The common types of medical emergencies that are most likely to happen are listed below:

- Fainting (syncope), the most common
- Fainting during sedation
- Anaphylactic shock
- Diabetic hypoglycaemic
- Epileptic attack
- Cardiac arrest
- Stroke
- Shock
- Choking or difficulty with breathing
- Asthmatic attack
- Haemorrhage
- Burns/scalds

Minimise the risk

Emergencies must be eliminated where possible; it is far better to avoid the occurrence than have to deal with it; the risk can be minimised in a variety of ways:

Reception
- Create a relaxed and pleasant atmosphere environmentally and personally.
- Be aware of patients' apprehensions and communicate effectively to alleviate any fears.
- Give the patient your full attention.

Surgery
- Ensure surgery is well ventilated.
- Talk to the patient and give a brief explanation of the dental procedure.
- Ask the patient to remove heavy outer clothing.
- Check and update medical history.
- Ensure that preoperative instructions have been followed.
- Allow the patient to stop and interrupt the procedure.
- Observe and reassure the patient throughout.
- Provide efficient chair side support, for example, protect soft tissues, aspirate carefully and respond to patient's needs.
- Observe the patient and be responsive to changes in his/her condition.
- Ensure that all post-operative instructions are given both verbally and in writing.
- Do not allow the patient to leave until he or she is fit to do so.

The whole of the dental team can be part of this procedure, which starts when the patient enters the reception area and is greeted by the receptionist and terminates when he/she is dismissed from the practice on the instruction of the dentist.

Managing medical emergencies

It is not always possible to eliminate an emergency even if you have carried out all procedures to minimise the risk. The dental team must be prepared to act if an emergency situation arises; a well-planned rehearsed routine saves lives. The dental setting should have an emergency drug kit that consists of the following *(Source: Resuscitation Council (UK) revised June 2008)*:

- **Emergency drug kit**
  - □ Portable oxygen cylinder (D size) with pressure reduction valve and flow meter
  - □ Oxygen face mask with tubing
  - □ Basic set of oropharyngeal airways (sizes 1, 2, 3 and 4)
  - □ Pocket mask with oxygen port
  - □ Self-inflating bag and mask apparatus with oxygen reservoir and tubing (1-l size bag)
  - □ Variety of well-fitting adult and child face masks for attaching to self-inflating bag
  - □ Portable suction with appropriate suction catheters and tubing, for example, the Yankauer sucker
  - □ Single-use sterile syringes and needles
  - □ 'Spacer' device for inhaled bronchodilators
  - □ Automated blood glucose measurement device
  - □ Automated external defibrillator (AED)
  - □ For practices carrying out sedation – suction catheter sizes 6 and 10 French gauge (FG)

All staff must be familiar with the location of the equipment and it must be easily accessible. The location of the AED should be clearly marked with the UK Standard sign, rectangular in shape, white pictogram and text on a green background.

- **Preparation**
  - □ Emergency information is to be readily available.
  - □ Information is to be immediately accessible, placed next to telephone.
  - □ Emergency information includes emergency numbers/services, name, address, telephone number of practice, other useful numbers, that is, doctor and hospital.

- **Staff training**
  - □ All the team to be trained
  - □ Training updated routinely
  - □ Basic first aid and cardiopulmonary resuscitation (CPR) mandatory
  - □ Dental team to be competent to manage emergency situations

- **Emergency routine**
  - □ The team should establish routine and document.
  - □ Define specific roles in event of emergency.
  - □ Named person should be responsible for locating emergency kit.
  - □ Ensure emergency kit is accessible.

- **Practise emergency routine**
  - □ Practise regularly, 3 to 4 times a year.
  - □ Ensure staff are aware of and capable of specific roles.
  - □ Ensure that staff competently work as a team.

- **Emergency drug kit**
  - □ Store kit where it is readily available and easily accessible.
  - □ Appointed/trained person is responsible for kit.
  - □ Check supplies routinely, for example, expiry dates.
  - □ Maintain record of contents.
  - □ Replace used drugs immediately.

- **Patient observation**
  - □ Observe patient condition throughout treatment.
  - □ Be able to recognise vital signs, for example, pallor, breathing difficulties, pain.

Common emergencies

This section provides an overview of the most likely cause, signs and symptoms and action to be taken in each situation. It should be noted that from time to time opinions change; therefore, it is vitally important that the dental team keeps up to date with these changes.

Fainting (syncope)

The causes include reduced blood supply to the brain caused by anxiety, pain, hunger, fatigue, and high temperature.

- **Signs/symptoms**
  - □ Pale/clammy skin
  - □ Slow feeble pulse
  - □ Shivering

□ Sighing
□ Loss of consciousness
□ Heat
□ Thirst
□ Black and white vision
□ Dizziness
- Action
  □ Lower head and raise feet higher.
  □ Loosen tight clothing.
  □ Check pulse.
  □ If necessary, place in recovery position when casualty regains consciousness.
  □ Record all details on patient's medical history form.

Fainting during sedation

The causes are analgesic overdose, deficiency of oxygen and respiratory failure.

- Signs/symptoms
  □ Pale and clammy skin
  □ Feeble pulse
- Action
  □ Stop sedation immediately.
  □ Remove any obstructions from the mouth and clear airway.
  □ Administer oxygen.

Anaphylactic shock

The cause is severe allergic reaction to a drug or agent.

- Signs/symptoms
  □ Generalised itching and tingling
  □ Breathing difficulties
  □ Pale, cold and clammy skin
  □ Weak/rapid pulse
  □ Convulsions
- Action
  □ Lay the patient flat.
  □ Dentist administers intramuscular (IM) adrenaline, intravenous (IV) hydrocortisone, IM chlorpheniramine and oxygen.
  □ Call ambulance.
  □ Observe patient's airway as fluid can collect in the larynx causing swelling.
  □ If the patient's condition deteriorates and there is complete loss of blood pressure and/or no pulse present, administer CPR.

Diabetic hypoglycaemia

Diabetic hypoglycaemia is caused when blood sugar level falls below normal.

- Signs/symptoms
  □ Sudden onset
  □ Profuse sweating
  □ Aggressive/excitable/irritable/restless
  □ Rapid feeble pulse
  □ Headache
  □ Sweet smell on breath
  □ Palpitations
- Action
  □ Lay the patient flat.
  □ Administer sugar orally.
  □ If patient looses consciousness the dentist administers IV glucose.

Epileptic attack

Causes include various factors such as hereditary, accident, injury during birth, severe infection and high fever causing damage.

- Signs/symptoms
- Initial stage
  □ Aura phase
    • Irritable, headache
- Second stage
  □ Tonic phase
    • Spasms, loss of consciousness
- Third stage
  □ Clonic phase
    • Uncontrolled jerking, convulsions
- Action
  □ Protect patient from hurting themselves.
  □ Move all equipment out of the way.
  □ Protect patient's head.
  □ Observe breathing and check pulse.
  □ If fit does not stop after few minutes the dentist administers IV diazepam and oxygen; call ambulance.

Cardiac arrest

See section on basic life support.
  The causes include severe hypotension, myocardial infarction and oxygen deficiency.

- Signs/symptoms
  □ The skin of the patient may be pale/clammy and may have a grey complexion.

□ Pulse is weak or absent.
□ There may be shortness of breath.
□ Patient may feel nauseous and could vomit.
□ There may be loss of consciousness.
□ The patient may develop severe crushing pain across the chest, radiating across the front of the chest and into the neck, shoulders and the left arm.

■ Action
□ Assess the patient and summon ambulance immediately.
□ Support patient's back and head with pillows, allow him/her to rest in a comfortable position.
□ Have suction ready in case of vomiting.
□ Administer high flow of oxygen, aspirin and, where the patient is not in shock, glyceryl trinitrate (GTN).
□ Have AED close by and ready.
□ Be prepared to administer CPR if trained to required level.
□ When ambulance service arrives, inform of all treatment and medication administered and provide the same in writing.

Stroke

The causes are sudden interruption in the blood supply to the brain, ruptured blood vessels, thrombosis and hypertension.

■ Signs/symptoms
□ Loss of consciousness
□ Weakness of arm and/or leg on one side causing partial paralysis
□ Partial paralysis on one side of face causing it to droop
■ Action
□ Call the ambulance immediately.
□ Keep airway clear.
□ Keep patient in horizontal position, with the head raised, and support the body.
□ Dentist administers oxygen.

Shock

Causes include loss of body fluids, that is, haemorrhage, hypotension, bacterial infection in the bloodstream, anaphylaxis or emotional shock.

■ Signs/symptoms
Similar to those of fainting, plus the following:
□ Dry mouth
□ Dilated pupils
□ Reduced flow of urine
■ Action
□ Call ambulance immediately.
□ Keep patient warm.

Choking/difficulty with breathing

Causes include obstruction by an inhaled object, for example, endodontic instrument, fragment of tooth or filling material.

■ Sign/symptoms
□ The patient is having difficulty with breathing.
□ Patient is choking.
■ Action
□ Encourage patient to cough.
□ Try to remove with the aspirator.
□ Give several sharp blows between the shoulder blades.
□ If all the above fails, the dentist performs the **Heimlich Manoeuvre** by standing behind the casualty and placing hands between the naval and rib cage and performing a sudden thrust.
□ Refer patient to hospital for chest X-ray.

Asthmatic attack

Causes include anxiety, infection and allergic reaction.

■ Signs/symptoms
□ Wheezing
□ Difficulty with breathing
□ Tightness in the chest
□ Patient appearing anxious
■ Action
□ Instruct patient to use his/her own medication, that is, salbutamol inhaler.
□ Calm the patient and encourage him/her to relax.
□ In severe cases, the dentist administers IV hydrocortisone and oxygen.
□ Call ambulance.

Haemorrhage

The cause is usually associated with extraction of a tooth.

- Signs/symptoms
  - □ Profuse bleeding from the operation sight.
  - □ Bleeding continues to occur for a long period of time.
- Action
  - □ Place sterile pressure pad over the operation site; ask patient to bite firmly.
  - □ If bleeding persists, suturing may be required to hold the tissues together.

Burns/scalds

Causes include direct contact with the flame from a Bunsen burner, handling a hot dry instrument, spillage of a chemical substance onto the skin or steam from the autoclave.

- Signs/symptoms
  - □ Redness, swelling and blistering of the skin.
  - □ May be painful.
  - □ If there is peeling or skin looks charred or grey, but not painful, it may be deep and serious.
- Action
  - □ If possible, remove any constricting items, that is, rings, watches or clothing before swelling occurs.
  - □ Cool the area under slow running water for 10 minutes or longer, if pain continues.
  - □ Cover the burn with sterile dressing.
  - □ If signs/symptoms appear deep and serious cover burn and refer to hospital.

The purpose of emergency aid in any of the above-mentioned types of emergencies is to preserve life, prevent the condition from worsening and promote recovery.

Basic life support (BLS)

In the event of a medical emergency and if the patient has collapsed, the general CPR guidelines/principles of the Resuscitation Council (UK) should be applied as follows *(Source:*

Resuscitation Council (UK) Cardiopulmonary Resuscitation – Standards for Clinical Practice and Training) (revised June 2008):

Follow the **A.B.C.D.E.** approach to assess and treat the patient:

- **Airway** – look for signs of airway obstruction, clear the airway, give oxygen at a high inspired concentration.
- **Breathing** – diagnose and treat life-threatening breathing problems immediately.
- **Circulation** – assess the likely causes and respond accordingly.
- **Disability** – review and treat the A.B.C., determine the cause and level of unconsciousness and treat immediately.
- **Exposure** – loosen or remove clothing to check patient for any rashes or oedema and avoid heat loss.

Adult basic life support

The priority for BLS is to deliver chest compressions, which consist of the following sequence of actions:

- Make sure the victim, any bystanders, and you are safe. Check the victim for a response.
- Gently shake his/her shoulders and ask loudly, 'Are you all right?' If there is no response, shout for help.
- Turn the casualty onto his/her back and then open the airway using head tilt and chin lift. Place your hand on his/her forehead and gently tilt the head back. With your fingertips under the point of the casualty's chin, lift the chin to open the airway.
- Keeping the airway open, look, listen, and feel for normal breathing.
  - □ Look for chest movement.
  - □ Listen at the victim's mouth for breath sounds.
  - □ Feel for air on your cheek.

  In the first few minutes after cardiac arrest, a casualty may be barely breathing, or taking infrequent and noisy gasps. Do not confuse this with normal breathing. Look, listen, and feel for no more than 10 seconds to determine if the casualty is breathing normally. If you have any doubt whether breathing is normal, act as if it is not normal.

- If they are not breathing normally, ask someone to call for an ambulance or, if you are on your own, do this yourself; you may need to leave the casualty. Start chest compression as follows:
  - □ Kneel by the side of the casualty.
  - □ Place the heel of one hand in the centre of the casualty's chest.
  - □ Place the heel of your other hand on top of the first hand.
  - □ Interlock the fingers of your hands and ensure that pressure is not applied over the casualty's ribs. Do not apply any pressure over the upper abdomen or the bottom end of the bony sternum (breastbone).
  - □ Position yourself vertically above the casualty's chest and, with your arms straight, press down on the sternum 4 to 5 cm.
  - □ After each compression, release all the pressure on the chest without losing contact between your hands and the sternum.
  - □ Repeat at a rate of about 100 times a minute (a little less than 2 compressions a second). Compression and release should take an equal amount of time.
- Combine chest compression with rescue breaths. After 30 compressions open the airway again using head tilt and chin lift.
  - □ Pinch the soft part of the victim's nose closed, using the index finger and thumb of your hand on his/her forehead.
  - □ Allow the mouth to open, but maintain chin lift.
  - □ Take a normal breath and place your lips around his mouth, making sure that you have a good seal.
  - □ Blow steadily into his mouth whilst watching for his chest to rise; take about 1 second to make his chest rise as in normal breathing; this is an effective rescue breath (approximately two ventilations)
  - □ Maintaining head tilt and chin lift, take your mouth away from the victim and watch for his chest to fall as air comes out.
  - □ Take another normal breath and blow into the victim's mouth once more to give a total

of two effective rescue breaths. Then return your hands without delay to the correct position on the sternum and give 30 more chest compressions.
  - □ Continue with chest compressions and rescue breaths in a ratio of 30:2.
- Continue resuscitation until
  - □ qualified help arrives and takes over;
  - □ the victim starts breathing normally; or
  - □ you become exhausted.

The above-mentioned BLS is performed when there is no equipment available, for example, an AED. It is unlikely BLS will revive a casualty if used as a stand-alone procedure. The Resuscitation Council (UK) recommends that an AED be used as part of the above to greatly enhance the chance of survival.

Summary

Ensure that patient medical history is reviewed at each and every appointment; ask the patient if there have been any changes since the last time they attended. Time is critical in any emergency situation; therefore, the dental team must have a well-practised routine to ensure that emergencies are managed effectively and efficiently to preserve life. Do not attempt to administer first aid or emergency aid unless you have been trained to do so. Ensure that you receive adequate and appropriate training frequently in order for you to provide competent assistance in the event of an emergency and record the training. Dental professionals are required to receive regular training in medical emergencies as laid down by the General Dental Council as one of the mandatory continuing professional development (CPD) core topics and the training should be recorded (Figure 14.1).

All emergencies and accidents must be entered into the accident 'book'. They must be investigated and analysed in line with the significant event analysis procedures and records held in accordance with the Data Protection Act.

Figure 14.1 Medical emergencies training log.

In column 3 'Specific topic' please record the medical emergency training you have received; a list of topics can be found below.

Name	Job title	Specific topic	Date	Signature

Medical emergencies: specific topics

1. Fainting
2. Diabetic hypoglycaemic
3. Cardiac arrest (CPR)
4. Shock
5. Asthmatic attack
6. Burns/scalds

7. Anaphylactic shock
8. Epileptic attack
9. Stroke
10. Choking or difficulty in breathing
11. Haemorrhage
12. Other (please specify)

Action – check the following

- Is the emergency drugs kit maintained and do you have a named person responsible for it?
- Have all staff received training in the emergencies mentioned in this chapter and has training been recorded?
- Are individuals competent to manage emergency situations and do you practise the procedure regularly to ensure effective and efficient team management?

Frequently asked questions

Q. What is the purpose of an automated external defibrillator (AED)?

A. An AED interprets a person's heart rhythm and determines if an electric shock is needed to stabilise the rhythm of the heart. The AED has an in-built mechanism which will not deliver the shock unless it is required. The Resuscitation Council (UK) recommends that an AED should be part of the emergency equipment in all dental settings.

Q. Does a person have to be qualified to use an AED?

A. The annual medical emergencies' training which all dental personnel must undertake should include the use of AEDs. The equipment is relatively easy to operate as it provides step-by-step verbal or visual instructions for the user to follow. It is important that this person is able to interpret basic instructions and information and is aware of the safety issues associated with its use. At the time of writing, there is no requirement for a formal qualification.

Q. Is there any risk of contracting an infection through mouth-to-mouth ventilation?

A. Although the risk is unlikely, precautions should be taken to reduce the possibility, for example, the use of a mask is advisable. It is reported that the following diseases could be transmitted *(Source: Arend, Carlos Frederico. Transmission of Infectious Diseases through mouth to mouth ventilation: evidence-based or emotion-based medicine.)*:

☐ Tuberculosis
☐ Herpes simplex
☐ Meningitis
☐ *Salmonella*

No cases of hepatitis or human immunodeficiency virus (HIV) have been reported.

Links to other chapters

Chapter 1 – Accidents and first aid

15 Occupational health and well-being

Scope of this chapter

- Introduction
- Legislation
- Definition
- Causes of ill health
- Managing the health and well-being of employees
- Support mechanisms
- Benefits to the business

Figures

Introduction

People spend 60% of their waking hours at work; employers fail to promote good health and the British workforce is unhealthy. During 2007–2008, 29 million working days were lost through ill health, of which 16 million was due to physical ill health and 13 million due to mental ill health. Lifestyles have changed over the last two decades, resulting in what is commonly termed *lifestyle diseases*. These are diseases brought about by the relationship between people and their environment, for example, those associated with diet, alcohol consumption, smoking, drug abuse and different life stressors. These types of diseases are chronic in nature and can be very difficult to cure; however, they are preventable. Over the last 25 years, life expectancy has increased considerably. In 1980–1982 life expectancy for men was approximately 72 years and for women 77 years. Compare this with figures for 2005–2007 where the life expectancy for men is 77 years and for women 82 years. It is a fact that people are living longer. In 2007, the number of older people in Great Britain was higher than the number under the age of 16 years. Combine this with the recently implemented age discrimination laws and what this shows is that we have an ageing workforce. However, this workforce is not necessarily in good health or free from illness *(Source: National Statistics)*. The above evidence highlights the need for employers to ensure the health and well-being of their workforce and that this is as much a priority as is their safety. This will not only demonstrate a commitment to employees but also have financial benefits for the business by reducing sickness and absence. Employers can help improve the health and well-being of their workforce by actively investing in workplace initiatives that promote good health.

Legislation

■ Health and Safety at Work etc. Act 1974:

Employers have a general duty to ensure, so far as is reasonably possible, the health, safety and welfare of all employees. The general duty covers the physical and psychological well-being of employees and the individual needs of each employee should be considered.

■ Management of Health and Safety at Work Regulations 1999:

Employers to make suitable and sufficient assessments of risks to health and safety of employees to identify the measures needed to remove the risks or reduce to an acceptable level. This includes controlling workplace risks by investing in their health and well-being.

■ Working Time Regulations 1998 (as amended):

Excessive working hours are a contributory factor to a person's health and well-being. Employers must organise and manage working hours to enable employees to maintain a healthy and fulfilling work life balance.

■ Employment Equality (Age) Regulations 2006:

Older employees must be provided with the same health and well-being opportunities, including statutory sick pay, in the same way as other employees.

Definition

Quite simply, occupational health and well-being is a combination of physical, social, intellectual and emotional fitness of 'people associated with work'. The range of people associated with work includes the existing workforce, new employees and those returning to work following a period of absence. Employers should therefore consider all groups when devising health and well-being programmes. It is understood that if a person is happy, contented and comfortable with their life, then they will be in good health and this is what employers should be aiming to achieve when devising programmes.

Causes of ill health

Mortality rates and lifestyles are important factors to consider when determining causes of ill health. These alone have brought about significant changes in society which have a direct impact on the health and well-being of employees. In addition, the following factors are particularly relevant and need to be considered by employers:

■ Safety
  □ Unsafe working practices
  □ Poor ergonomic workplace design
  □ Ineffective accident/significant event analysis procedure
  □ No assessment of health risks
  □ Inadequate infection control procedures
  □ Lack of safety and health awareness training
  □ Poor safety culture
■ Environmental
  □ Inefficient and inappropriate heating
  □ Lack of natural light and unsuitable artificial lighting
  □ Poor ventilation
  □ Uncontrolled management of waste
  □ Poor housekeeping
■ Organisational and professional
  □ Unachievable targets
  □ Advances in technology
  □ Working times and patterns
  □ Change process
  □ Unworkable policies
  □ Customer demands and expectations
  □ Professional requirements

- Management style
  - ☐ Autocratic
  - ☐ Unapproachable
  - ☐ Poor communication
  - ☐ Ineffective leadership
  - ☐ Poor resource management
  - ☐ Blame culture

The above-mentioned factors can have a detrimental effect on the health and well-being of employees. All are preventable and should be analysed as part of the management health and well-being programme.

Managing the health and well-being of employees

The government review, *Working for a Healthier Tomorrow*, undertaken by Dame Carol Black and published in 2008, showed that the health of people of working age must be high on the agenda for all businesses. For an occupational health and well-being programme to be successful it must have the involvement and commitment of employers and employees. It will require the allocation of resources, changes in attitudes and behaviours and support from both internal and external parties.

Employers

The overall responsibility for establishing how to minimise the likelihood of people becoming ill and for making the health and well-being programme work lies with the employer. There are a range of initiatives that should be considered:

- Understand the needs of employees to enable a balance of work and personal issues.
- Develop flexible policies and look for opportunities to meet employee and organisational needs.
- Review and implement health, well-being and sickness absence policies and procedures.
- Ensure that the workplace is safe and environmentally healthy, as far as is reasonable.

- Carry out pre-employment medical screening to identify existing conditions which you will need to consider when allocating work.
- Identify the need for health surveillance programmes.
- Implement workplace health promotion programmes for employees.
- Organise work effectively and consider working hours and systems of work.
- Identify causes of ill health; eliminate or reduce the risks.
- Take time out of work for team-building activities.
- Support staff who return to work after illness by considering changing work patterns or making workplace adaptations.
- Train managers in human resource management and in how to deal effectively with sickness absence and return to work discussions.
- Consider the government's new 'fit note' sickness certification programme and how the proposed three categories of ability to work can be implemented:
  - ☐ Fit for work
  - ☐ Not fit for work
  - ☐ May be fit for some work now
- Invest in and work with other health-care professionals and use support mechanisms.
- Be aware of current epidemics and pandemics and put appropriate measures in place to prevent the spread of infection.
- Encourage open consultation and communication with employees.

Assess how well you are meeting the needs of your employees and identify areas for development (Figure 15.1).

Employees

Employees have a responsibility to cooperate with the employer in the programme and to maintain their own health. They should

- assess their lifestyles and reflect on what is having a detrimental effect;
- strike a happy balance between work and personal life;

- eat a well-balanced diet, having the 'sins' in moderation;
- reduce alcohol consumption and other habits that could affect physical health;
- avoid or defuse harmful and stressful situations;
- take time out to relax and get fit;
- have a periodic health check and fitness assessment;
- do regular mind and body exercises;
- take part in team exercises;
- discuss concerns, issues and problems with managers/employers and aim to resolve them;

- participate in consultation processes on policies and procedures which affect their working lives;
- have control over their pace of work and ensure they have the skills and abilities to perform safely;
- seek medical advice if they suspect their health and well-being is at risk.

Employees should be encouraged to reflect on lifestyles and identify areas that may need reviewing in order to achieve work–life balance (Figure 15.2).

Figure 15.1 Employer organisational questionnaire.

This questionnaire is designed to help your organisation to measure how well it is supporting employees to achieve occupational health and well-being.

The highest score is 45.

1 = NO   2 = Working towards   3 = Yes

1. Does your organisation acknowledge that individuals work best when they can achieve a balance between work and personal life?   3   2   1

2. Does your organisation recognise that work–life balance will benefit the business?   3   2   1

3. Does your organisation communicate health and well-being to employees?   3   2   1

4. Does your organisation encourage employees to discuss difficulties in achieving work–life balances?   3   2   1

5. Does your organisation train managers in the benefits of implementing flexible working policies?   3   2   1

6. Do you take time out for away day team-building activities?   3   2   1

7. Does your organisation value people for their contribution to the business?   3   2   1

8. Does your organisation offer a range of flexible working options, that is, part-time, job share, etc.?   3   2   1

9. Does your organisation survey staff opinions about how they would like to work more effectively?   3   2   1

10. Does your organisation have systems in place to manage safety and environmental issues?   3   2   1

11. Do you have an open and honest policy to listen to staff?   3   2   1

12. Do you annually review your working arrangements in the organisation?   3   2   1

13. Do you have a structured training and development process?   3   2   1

14. Is your organisation up to date with legislative requirements, that is, working time regulations, flexible working provisions etc.?   3   2   1

15. Do you evaluate and monitor change that may affect your business?   3   2   1

Total score:

Do you need to improve occupational health and well-being throughout the organisation?   Yes   No

Figure 15.2   Employee health and well-being questionnaire.

This questionnaire is designed to help you, the employee, to measure how well you are maintaining your own health and well-being in order to achieve the work–life balance.

The highest score is 45.

1 = NO   2 = Working towards   3 = Yes

1. I sleep at least 6 hours every night	3	2	1
2. I eat three nutritions meals a day	3	2	1
3. I drink alcohol in moderation	3	2	1
4. I eat only healthy snacks	3	2	1
5. I stay away from harmful and stressful situations	3	2	1
6. I put aside at least 2 hours a night to relax	3	2	1
7. I thoroughly enjoy my job	3	2	1
8. I get a lot of satisfaction from my home life	3	2	1
9. I am a very happy person and smile a lot	3	2	1
10. I am totally content with my inner-self	3	2	1
11. I am a very positive thinker (glass is always half full)	3	2	1
12. I look at myself in the mirror and like what I see	3	2	1
13. I walk or exercise at least three times a week	3	2	1
14. I have had a complete health check in the last 2 years	3	2	1
15. My blood pressure and cholesterol count are normal and my weight is in the ideal range	3	2	1

Total score:

Do you need to take action to improve your health and well-being in order to achieve the work–life balance?   Yes   No

Support mechanisms

There are a range of organisations that can provide support and help influence effective health and well-being programmes and some of these are listed below. Employers will need to assess their level of need and the organisations that are most appropriate.

Occupational health

The aim of the service is to prevent and minimise health-related illness and risks in the workplace. It achieves this by providing the following services:

- Treating medical emergencies at work
- Conducting pre-employment health examinations
- Conducting pre-placement health examinations to assess fitness against specific job roles
- Identifying areas of activity where health surveillance is required, that is, immunisation and mercury screening
- Carrying out health surveillance on persons exposed to specific health hazards
- Advising on fitness of employees for monitoring those on work restrictions, that is, expectant mothers
- Advising on fitness of employees during long-term absence and on return to work

- Participating in managing treatment and rehabilitation of employees to aid recovery
- Providing personal advice in health matters relating to work
- Providing health promotion and lifestyle advice to promote employee well-being
- Advising and assisting on relevant workplace assessments, for example, ergonomic assessments
- Maintaining confidential and appropriate records

Occupational health services are now taking a more proactive approach in preventing cases of ill health rather than only treating the outcome. Employers will need to determine what level of service is required and how it is to be provided. At the time of writing, those who have a National Health Service (NHS) dental contract in England have access to an occupational health service.

Other health care/health and safety professionals

A range of other organisations that can all have a role in helping employers shape their health and well-being programme are listed below:

- Health promotion agencies
- General medical practitioners and nurses
- Ergonomics experts (ergonomists)
- Trade unions
- Health and safety consultant/practitioners

Primary Care Trusts (PCTs) and Local Health Boards (LHBs)

Primary Care Trusts (PCTs) and Local Health Boards (LHBs) are able to provide information on business management issues in relation to the contract, in particular, advise on local strategies to meet the needs of patients. These strategies will have a direct effect on how the business is managed and the impact it will have on the team. In some cases, they may also be able to allocate resources to improve and develop the performance of the business, which, in turn, will enable employees to work more efficiently and effectively. PCTs may also organise seminars on health- and well-being-related issues for the dental team.

Department of Health (DH)

The Department of Health (DH) produces policy and guidance, publications, consultation documents and reports regarding government initiatives relating to healthy workplaces. A range of topics are readily available, including health care, social care, public health issues and information on how to manage your organisation.

Health and Safety Executive (HSE)

The primary function of the Health and Safety Executive (HSE) is to prevent death, injury and ill health to all those associated with work. This includes the workforce and anyone who may be affected. The HSE provides authoritative information and guidance on all aspects of health, safety, welfare and well-being.

World Health Organization (WHO)

The World Health Organization (WHO) provides leadership on global health issues and helps shape and influence the health research agenda, set standards, and disseminate information on changing trends in world health.

Benefits to the business

Being known as an organisation that cares about staff enhances an employer's reputation and can help attract staff and customers. In addition, the practice can benefit in other ways.

- Costs of sickness absence can be reduced.
- Simple measures to prevent and manage ill health can reduce absenteeism, which, in turn, improves productivity and competitive edge.
- Getting employees back into work after illness reduces the loss of experienced staff and the cost of recruiting new staff.
- Healthy working environments reduce employee absence through sickness and stress.
- Employees who feel cared for are more satisfied and perform better, therefore reducing staff turnover and increasing productivity.

Summary

Research shows that work is important for a person's health. It not only provides the resources to maintain a particular lifestyle but more importantly it helps to prevent ill health so that the fruits of the labour can be enjoyed. A healthy workforce is a sustainable workforce and so it is important that employees are in good health and feel good about themselves. Employers should ensure that employees are not injured or made ill at work, consider health and well-being during business planning and demonstrate that they care about their staff by promoting the healthy workplace.

Action – check the following

- Do you have a health and well-being policy that demonstrates your commitment to your staff?
- Do you have systems in place for individuals to raise concerns?
- Have you identified suitable and appropriate support mechanisms to assist with your programme?

Frequently asked questions

Q. What action should be taken if an employee refuses to participate in health screening/surveillance?

A. Taking action against a member of staff who refuses to participate in occupational health screening/surveillance is extremely difficult. However, it should first be managed by fully explaining the reason for such measures and emphasising that it is for the benefit of the employee to reduce all foreseeable risks. In addition, it should be included in the terms and conditions of employment as this will ensure that employees know they have to comply. Any changes to the employment contract must be made using the 90-day change period. Ultimately, the Health and Safety at Work etc. Act 1974 Section 7 states that employees have a duty to cooperate with their employer. This should be explained and agreed on when employees are recruited.

Q. Is the employer permitted to have access to occupational health records?

A. Occupational health records of employees belong to the employer and therefore should be kept in a secure format and not accessed by unauthorised persons.

Links to other chapters

Chapter 1 – Accidents and first aid
Chapter 2 – Alcohol, drugs and smoking
Chapter 4 – Conflict management
Chapter 9 – Hazardous substances
Chapter 11 – Lone working
Chapter 19 – Risk assessment
Chapter 20 – Stress management
Chapter 23 – Working environment
Chapter 24 – Working hours

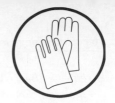

16 Personal protective equipment

Scope of this chapter

- Introduction
- Legislation
- Range of PPE and risk assessment
- Employer's responsibilities – the PPE/C process
- Employees' responsibilities

Figures

Figure 16.1 – PPE/C range and risk assessment.
Figure 16.2 – The PPE/C process.

Introduction

Personal protective equipment/clothing (PPE/C) is held or worn by an individual in order to protect against foreseeable risks to which he/she is exposed during the course of his/her work. It must only be provided where these risks cannot be **adequately** controlled by other means. For example, eye protection is worn to prevent debris splatter entering the eye during dental treatment procedures. The aspirator does not remove all particles at source; therefore, PPE is required as a last resort. PPE also includes clothing if the clothing is intended to protect against a foreseeable risk.

Legislation

- Personal Protective Equipment at Work Regulations 1992 (as amended 2002) (exceptions apply where marked*):

  Employers are required to select, provide and maintain suitable PPE and to ensure appropriate use, where risks cannot be adequately controlled by any other means.

- Health and Safety at Work etc. Act 1974:

  Employers are required to ensure, so far as is reasonably possible, the health, safety and welfare of all employees.

- Management of Health and Safety at Work Regulations 1999:

  Employers [are] to make suitable and sufficient assessments of risks to health and safety of employees to identify the measures needed to

Managing Health and Safety in the Dental Practice: A Practical Guide, by Jane Bonehill © 2010 by Blackwell Publishing Ltd.

remove the risks or reduce to an acceptable level.

- Control of Substances Hazardous to Health Regulations 2002* (exceptions apply):

  Requires employers to assess risks to health from exposure to hazardous substances by employees and prevent exposure where reasonably possible, where not possible to control exposure and protect health.

- The Control of Noise at Work Regulations 2005* (exceptions apply):

  Requires employers to prevent or reduce risks to health and safety from exposure to noise at work.

- Personal Protective Equipment Regulations 2002:

  Responsibilities are placed on designers, manufacturers and suppliers of PPE to ensure PPE complies with safety requirements and the European Union (EU) 'CE Mark' is clearly visible.

Range of PPE and risk assessment

Personal protection includes **equipment and clothing** (PPE/C) (Figure 16.1). In this chapter, it includes that which is relevant to dental practice; therefore, other items have been excluded as they are not relevant to the dental profession. Relevant items are as follows:

- Gloves
- Safety footwear
- Safety glasses
- Face shield
- Masks
- Visors
- Armlets
- Clinical clothing[1]

---

[1] This item may not be classed as PPE/C; however, if it is provided as a result of the risk assessment to protect against a foreseeable risk, then it comes under the definition.

- Aprons
- Ear protection[2]
- Barrier creams/hand hygiene products[3]

Employer's responsibilities – the PPE/C process

PPE is provided as a last resort. Therefore, in order to **determine the need (1)** for PPE/C, **risk assessments** must be undertaken on all relevant work activities. This will identify the hazards people are exposed to and how they are at risk. Figures 16.1 and 16.2 will help you decide which activities need to be assessed.

The next stage is to **select** the **appropriate PPE/C (2)** for the identified risk. Involve the users and consult with them in order to gain their opinion and to encourage their commitment.

Then **identify the characteristics (3)** of the PPE/C which are required to protect against identified risks; this should include the following:

- Does it protect from the risks identified?
- Is it well fitting and, if necessary, adjustable?
- Will it allow the users to move freely and undertake their work safely?
- If more than one item is required, are they compatible and do they protect against the risk – for example, where both safety glasses and a mask are worn?
- Will it allow for normal work activities to be undertaken to the required standard and not interfere with patient care?

PPE/C must not be provided without giving **information, instruction and training (4)** to users

---

[2] These items are not routinely provided; however, the risk assessment may identify the need to provide under exceptional circumstances in order to adequately control risks (see Figure 16.1 for further explnation).

[3] These are not classed as PPE and, therefore, do not come under the PPE Regulations; however, they are routinely used in dentistry to maintain the pH balance, keep skin healthy and protect from adverse reactions when wearing gloves.

Figure 16.1 PPE/C range and risk assessment.

Range	Protection	Characteristics	Procedure	Maintenance
Gloves – type 1 Examination/treatment gloves	Hand	• Well fitting for individual user • Powder free • Preferably latex free • Odourless and tasteless • Good wet and dry grip • Tactile sensitivity • Antibacterial	• All clinical procedures	• Dispose after each patient or if damaged • Remove before leaving clinical area
Gloves – type 2 Non-medical gloves	Hand	• Well fitting for individual user • Heavy duty strength and durability • Puncture and chemical resistant • Good hold and grip • Latex free • Rolled cuff • Allows manual dexterity	• Handling sharps, hot instruments and chemicals during decontamination procedures • Changing radiographic solutions	• Rinse in cold water and disinfect after single use • Store in clean, cool dry area away from direct sunlight • Check expiry date • Replace if damaged • Remove before leaving clinical area
Safety footwear	Feet	• Specific size for user • Toe area covered • Non-slip sole	• All clinical procedures • Using chemicals decontamination procedures • Handling sharps and hot instruments	• Regular examination to check condition • Replace if badly damaged or worn
Safety glasses	Eyes	• Well fitting for individual user • Light weight • Full, clear, antimist strengthened lenses and side protection • May be worn over glasses • Good optical quality • Compatible with mask • Protect from radiation emissions – laser wavelength	• All clinical procedures • Using chemicals during decontamination procedures • Changing radiographic solutions • Laser procedures	• Disinfected after each patient • Store away from risk of scratching • Replace when optical quality impaired • Remove before leaving clinical area
Face shield	Eyes	• Tinted shield covering eyes • Handle provides firm grip • Protect from radiation emissions, for example, curing lights	• Light curing procedures	• Disinfected after each patient • Store from risk of scratching • Replace when optical quality impaired

(*continued overleaf*)

Figure 16.1 (*continued*)

Range	Protection	Characteristics	Procedure	Maintenance
Masks	Nose and mouth	• Lightweight • Good filtration • Adjustable noseband • High breathability • Fluid resistant • Ear loops or tie on • Compatible with safety glasses	• All clinical procedures • Using chemicals during decontamination procedures	• Dispose after each patient or if heavily soiled • Remove before leaving clinical area
Visors	Eyes, nose and mouth	• Well fitting for individual user • Lightweight • Full, clear face covering and side protection • May be worn over glasses • Good optical quality	• All clinical procedures • Using chemicals during decontamination procedures	• Disinfect after each patient • Store away from risk of scratching • Replace when optical quality impaired • Remove before leaving clinical area
Armlets	Forearms	• Well fitting for individual user • Adjustable at flex area • Cuffed	• Clinical procedures in preference to arm hygiene routine • Changing radiographic solution • Decontamination procedures	• Remove and change after each patient • Wash separately at a minimum of 65°C • Replace when worn or heavily soiled • Remove before leaving clinical area
Clinical clothing	Body	• Well fitting for individual user • Flame retardant	• All clinical procedures • Decontamination procedures • Changing radiographic solutions	• Change daily or if heavily soiled • Wash separately at a minimum of 65°C • Replace when worn or heavily soiled • Remove before leaving practice
Aprons	Body; clinical clothing	• Splash proof • Disposable polythene	• Surgical procedures • Decontamination procedures • Changing radiographic solutions	• Dispose after each patient • Remove before leaving clinical area
*Ear protection	Ears	• Good speech recognition • Ergonomic design • Well fitting for individual user • Tapered soft foam • Lowest decibel reduction	• Clinical procedures when using high-speed handpiece & ultra sonic scaler	• Change after every session or if heavily contaminated • Remove when leaving clinical area

*Ear protection must not be provided as a first-line measure to reduce noise; noise must be controlled at source and ear protection provided only where the risk assessment deems it to be absolutely necessary to protect the individual user. The use of ear protection must not impair the communication process between patient, dental professional and other members of the team.

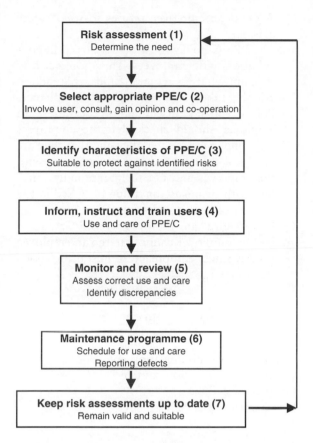

```
┌─────────────────────────────────┐
│      Risk assessment (1)         │◄──────┐
│      Determine the need          │       │
└─────────────────────────────────┘       │
              │                            │
              ▼                            │
┌─────────────────────────────────┐       │
│   Select appropriate PPE/C (2)   │       │
│ Involve user, consult, gain opinion and co-operation │
└─────────────────────────────────┘       │
              │                            │
              ▼                            │
┌─────────────────────────────────┐       │
│ Identify characteristics of PPE/C (3) │  │
│ Suitable to protect against identified risks │
└─────────────────────────────────┘       │
              │                            │
              ▼                            │
┌─────────────────────────────────┐       │
│ Inform, instruct and train users (4) │   │
│      Use and care of PPE/C       │       │
└─────────────────────────────────┘       │
              │                            │
              ▼                            │
┌─────────────────────────────────┐       │
│    Monitor and review (5)        │       │
│   Assess correct use and care    │       │
│     Identify discrepancies       │       │
└─────────────────────────────────┘       │
              │                            │
              ▼                            │
┌─────────────────────────────────┐       │
│  Maintenance programme (6)       │       │
│   Schedule for use and care      │       │
│       Reporting defects          │       │
└─────────────────────────────────┘       │
              │                            │
              ▼                            │
┌─────────────────────────────────┐       │
│ Keep risk assessments up to date (7) │───┘
│     Remain valid and suitable    │
└─────────────────────────────────┘
```

Figure 16.2   The PPE/C process.

on its use and care. This should include the following:

- Why it has been provided and the risks it will protect against
- How it will protect the user against the identified risks
- When and how it must be used and its limitations
- When and how it must be cleaned/decontaminated
- When it must be removed and replaced
- How it must be stored and disposed of
- The consequences of not adhering to the above

The use of PPE/C needs to be **monitored and reviewed** (5) to assess if it is being used, cleaned,

replaced, stored and disposed of correctly in line with the practice policy and to the manufacturer's requirements. In addition, monitoring will help identify any discrepancies with the existing system and changes that need to be made.

Most of the PPE/C provided in the dental practice is disposable. However, a **maintenance programme** (6) should state when it has to be removed, cleaned/decontaminated, replaced, stored or disposed of and should ensure that an efficient stock control system is in place and that replacements are always available. The programme should also include a reporting procedure if the PPE/C is defective.

Just like all other risk assessments, the PPE/C assessment **must be kept up to date** (7) to ensure that it remains valid and suitable. You should state in your policy when the provision of PPE/C will be reviewed.

Employees' responsibilities

Employees have a legal responsibility to apply the training received, which includes the following:

- Use or wear PPE/C which has been provided to protect the employees from identified risks.
- Care for it including cleaning/decontamination, removal, replacement, storage and disposal.
- Report any problems and defects.

Employers must take all steps to ensure that employees comply with the policy and use PPE/C as specified. If an employee refuses to comply he/she is liable for prosecution.

Summary

PPE/C must only be provided as a last resort, after a risk assessment has been undertaken to determine the need and suitability. It will only protect the individual user/wearer and not those in the immediate vicinity. Therefore, the effectiveness of the protection it provides is totally reliant on the cooperation of the user.

Action – check the following

- Have you provided PPE/C as a 'last resort' after carrying out a risk assessment, which identified the need?
- Does the PPE/C carry the EU 'CE Mark'?
- Have you provided sufficient information, instruction and training to employees on the use and care of PPE/C?
- Do you monitor and review the use of PPE/C to check compliance with the policy?
- Do you review the provision of PPE/C periodically?

Frequently asked questions

Q. Why is PPE/C provided as a 'last resort'?

A. PPE/C will not remove or eliminate the hazards and risks; therefore they still remain. It is provided where the risk assessment shows that the risks cannot be suitably controlled without providing PPE/C.

Q. What if an employee refuses to wear safety glasses?

A. The PPE/C policy must be developed in consultation with employees. This should clearly explain what is required and what action will be taken in cases of non-compliance. Before starting disciplinary procedures, an employer should check that the employees fully understands the policy and that they are aware of their legal duties to cooperate with the employer and not to intentionally interfere with or misuse anything provided in the interest of health and safety.

Q. Can I charge an employee for PPE/C?

A. No, an employer cannot charge an employee for any safety equipment. It must be provided free of charge.

Links to other chapters

Chapter 3 – Communication and training
Chapter 10 – Infection control
Chapter 17 – Policy
Chapter 19 – Risk assessment

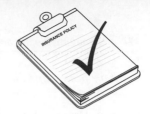

17 Policy

Scope of this chapter

Figures

Introduction

It is strongly advised that you read this chapter in conjunction with Chapter 12 in order to develop the Health and Safety Policy.

All dental establishments, regardless of the size or number of people employed, must have a policy for managing health and safety. Where five or more people are employed at any one time, the policy must be in writing. The policy must be brought to the attention of all employees and reviewed and revised as and when necessary. A clearly defined policy that is used in the day-to-day operations of the organisation assists employers in complying with legislation and maintaining workplace standards. In addition, it demonstrates the commitment of the employer to the health, safety and welfare of all persons who might be affected. Employers are required to consult with their staff prior to implementing or revising a policy; this provides the opportunity for people to discuss, seek advice and take an active part in ensuring that the policy is workable.

Legislation

- Health and Safety at Work etc. Act 1974:

  Requires employers, who employ 5 or more people, to prepare and as often as may be appropriate, revise their written health and safety policy and bring the statement and any revisions to the notice of all employees.

■ Employers Health and Safety Policy Statement (Exception) Regulations 1975:

Employers who employ less than 5 people at any one time are exempt from the requirement to have a written health and safety policy.

■ Management of Health and Safety at Work Regulations 1999:

Requires employers to arrange for the effective planning, organisation, control, monitoring and review of health and safety measures. Where 5 or more are employed these must be documented.

■ The Health and Safety (Consultation with Employees Regulations) 1996:

Requires employers to consult with employees when health and safety arrangements are formulated, implemented, monitored and reviewed.

■ The Information and Consultation of Employees Regulations 2004:

Requires employers of larger organisations, where more than 50 people are employed, to make or amend arrangements to inform and consult the workforce on issues which affect them.

Purpose of the policy

Health and safety in the dental practice needs to be managed, and the process must be structured, factual and tangible. The policy should influence all activities, including recruitment and selection of staff and all working methods. It should be reviewed and revised as and when appropriate and the revisions brought to the attention of all employees and other interested parties. The policy should consist of a series of documents that clearly state what the practice's aim is and how the practice intends to achieve the aim. This should be done through a series of objectives, to ensure the health, safety and welfare of all employees and non-employees. These documents should be 'user friendly', practical and specifically tailored to your practice needs; the individual documents will formulate the practice's Health and Safety Policy.

Preparing the policy

Step 1

When preparing your Health and Safety Policy for the first time, it is helpful to reflect on the working arrangements and procedures that you already have in place. This will help you determine if they are being carried out to an acceptable professional standard (Figure 17.1).

Step 2

The next stage is to set a clear aim and a series of objectives, covering the working arrangements and procedures, which state your commitment to health, safety and welfare. You will need to decide and agree on individual roles and responsibilities – everyone must have a responsibility; however, this will vary throughout the organisation and is usually dependent on seniority and competence. When deciding on who is going to do what, you must ensure that the person is trained and competent to fulfil that role and that he/she is in agreement with undertaking that role and you may need to provide training. The practice owner/most senior person will have overall responsibility. The day-to-day implementation of the policy could be delegated to the practice manager but accountabilities cannot be delegated! You are now ready to specify the arrangements to manage health and safety within your practice.

Step 3

Give your team the opportunity to consult on the draft document, distribute copies, set a timescale for feedback and collate comments.

Step 4

Make any necessary changes; this will not only ensure that the policy works for you but it also shows you to value your team's commitment. Your policy is now finalised and ready to be

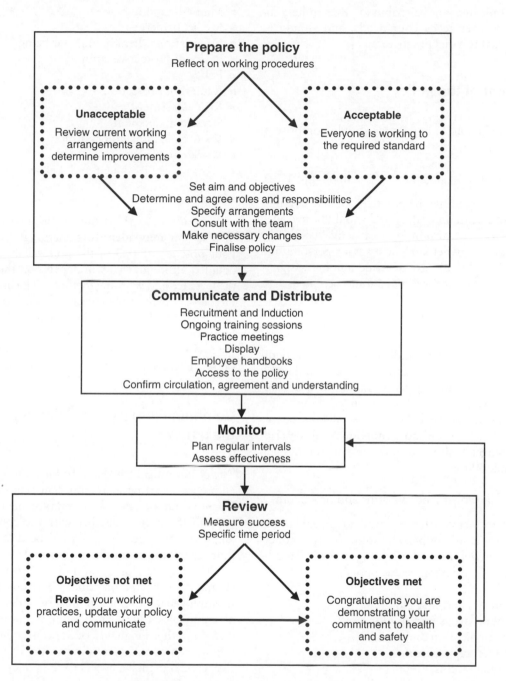

Figure 17.1 The Health and Safety Policy process.

communicated and distributed. Remember, the policy is specific to your needs, and should be individual to your practice.

Content of the policy

The Health and Safety Policy should comprise of three parts:

Part 1 – general statement of intent (Figure 17.2)

This should outline the practice's overall commitment to health and safety and should be specified in the form of an aim and objectives signed by the practice owner/s or most senior person/s and the policy should have an issue number assigned for updating purposes and should be dated.

Part 2 – organisation (roles and responsibilities) (Figure 17.3)

This should clearly indicate who is accountable and for whom and for what, and what the chain of authority is. It should also demonstrate how accountabilities are fixed, how policy implementation is to be monitored how people are to function and how individual job descriptions reflect health and safety responsibilities and accountabilities.

Part 3 – arrangements (systems and procedures)

This part details the practical arrangements in place to assist implementation of the policy. The following minimum arrangements should be included in a dental practice policy:

- Accidents and first aid
- Alcohol, drugs and smoking
- Communication and training
- Conflict management
- Disabled access
- Display screen equipment
- Electrical safety
- Fire safety and emergencies
- Hazardous substances
- Infection control
- Lone working
- Management systems

- Manual handling
- Medical emergencies
- Occupational health and well-being
- Personal protective equipment
- Policy
- Radiation protection
- Risk assessment
- Stress management
- Visitors, locums and contractors
- Work equipment
- Working environment and welfare
- Working hours

In addition to the above-mentioned arrangements, you may identify something specific to your practice. Part 3 of the policy may be quite detailed although this will depend on the size of the practice and working methods. The important factor is that the policy clearly states your commitment in each of the arrangements and explains how you are going to demonstrate your commitment (Refer individual chapters throughout this book to help specify the arrangements.).

Communicating and distributing the policy

The policy must be brought to the attention of all employees starting at recruitment (Figure 17.1). When you make an offer of employment, send a copy of the policy together with the contract of employment. The policy should be discussed in more detail at induction, and thereafter at ongoing training sessions and practice meetings. It should be displayed on notice boards or included in employee handbooks. It must be understood by all employees and this may require it to be reproduced in other languages or appropriate formats, taking into consideration individual capabilities. Everyone must have access to the policy and you need to decide the best method of bringing the policy to the attention of employees. You may choose to issue a complete copy to each person or a shortened version, but the full copy should be made available. You should confirm circulation, agreement to and understanding of the policy by asking employees to sign a declaration

Figure 17.2 Health and Safety Policy statement. (Example)

PRACTICE NAME AND NAME OF EMPLOYER/S: (insert details)

PRACTICE ADDRESS: (insert details)

ISSUE NUMBER: (e.g. 1)   **DATE:** (e.g. 02.01.2010)

The overall aim of our Health and Safety Policy is to ensure, so far as is reasonably possible, the health, safety and welfare of employees, non-employees and any one else who may be affected by our activities.

(Insert Name of Employer/s) recognises his/her duties under The Health and Safety at Work etc. Act 1974, European Regulations and professional requirements. This is demonstrated by complying with current legislation and adherence to best practice and through identifying and controlling risks.

The policy has been devised following consulting with the team in order to encourage commitment and ensure we meet our aim and objectives as stated below:

The practice will, so far as is reasonably possible:

1. Put arrangements and resources in place to effectively manage health and safety aimed at continually improving standards and business function.

2. Review the policy at planned intervals to identify any changes that affects the business function and revise as necessary.

3. Plan and implement a risk assessment programme in order to manage risks.

4. Provide appropriate information, instruction, training and supervision.

5. Provide and maintain a safe and healthy working environment.

6. Ensure universal precautions are adopted to prevent the spread of infection.

7. Reduce the risk of injury and ill health by providing suitable and sufficient personal protection.

8. Operate an accident reporting and recording system which includes investigating, analysing and preventing recurrence of all types of accidents.

9. Provide first aid facilities which are adequate and appropriate to the level of risk.

10. Ensure procedures are in place to identify all types of emergencies and provide suitable safety measures.

11. Identify hazardous substances and control the use, handling, storage, disposal and transportation.

12. Provide and maintain safe equipment and safe systems of work.

13. Prevent injuries resulting from moving and handling by assessing activities.

14. All activities involving the use of display screen equipment are assessed and suitably controlled.

15. Provide information for visitors, temporary staff and contractors.

16. Make reasonable access into and around the practice for disabled people.

17. Manage situations of conflict associated with internal and external customers.

18. Identify causes of stress, minimise risks and provide ongoing support.

19. Consider the safety of all persons who are working alone.

20. Have procedures in place to monitor behaviours and systems against set criteria.

21. Have effective consultation and communication methods in place which encourages the participation of all persons and provides opportunities to raise issues or concerns and develop safe working practices.

22. Identify and agree the duties and responsibilities of everyone.

23. Understanding of and agreement to the policy is required.

24. This statement is displayed to provide information for all interested parties.

SIGNED: (insert signature/s)   **EMPLOYER NAME/S:** (insert name/s)

DATE: (e.g. 02.01.2010)

Figure 17.3   Organisation (roles and responsibilities). (Example)

EMPLOYER: (insert name)

ACCOUNTABLE FOR: MANAGEMENT, COORDINATORS, EMPLOYEES AND NON-EMPLOYEES

- Assume overall responsibility for health and safety.
- Devise and implement a health and safety management system.
- Overall and final responsibility for preparing, implementing, monitoring, reviewing and revising the policy.
- Understand and keep up to date with the main requirements of legislation and its application to dental practice activities.
- Keep up to date with requirements for professional standards.
- Ensure the organisational structure is able to manage health and safety.
- To appoint competent persons to assist in the management of health and safety.
- Allocate sufficient and appropriate resources to manage health and safety.
- Demonstrate commitment and carry out safe working practices to provide direction for others.

PRACTICE MANAGER: (insert name)

ACCOUNTABLE TO: Employer

ACCOUNTABLE FOR: All employees and non-employees

- Understand in depth the Health and Safety Policy.
- Communicate and distribute the practice policy and procedures.
- Monitor and manage performance and behaviours of employees and non-employees in line with the policy.
- Monitor the effectiveness of the policy.
- Review and make recommendations to revise the policy.
- Allocate and agree roles and responsibilities and ensure people are competent to carry out their duties.
- Identify training needs, provide relevant training and maintain training records.
- Carry out inspections and risk assessments and make recommendations for improvement.
- Maintain health and safety records.
- Include health and safety in practice meetings and circulate minutes.
- Ensure the safe use and maintenance of all equipment.
- Ensure all accidents are recorded, investigated and acted upon.
- Ensure agreed methods of working are complied with.
- Review and revise the health and safety management system.

HEAD NURSE/NURSE COORDINATOR – (insert name)

ACCOUNTABLE TO: Practice manager

ACCOUNTABLE FOR: Dental nurses

- Provide suitable and appropriate supervision.
- Understand and comply with the Health and Safety Policy.
- Ensure correct working procedures are carried out and report any discrepancies.
- Assist with inducting new members of staff.
- Ensure nurses are adequately trained and informed.
- Identify training needs and source appropriate training provision.
- Assist in reviewing and revising working practices.
- Assist in accident reporting, investigation and prevention.
- Identify and report any hazardous situations, defective equipment and take immediate action to minimise the risk of injury.
- Take charge of first aid provision.

EMPLOYEES

ACCOUNTABLE TO: Practice manager

- Carry out all activities in line with the Health and Safety policy.
- Report unsafe acts and conditions.
- Use and maintain personal protective equipment/clothing.
- Use equipment and materials as instructed in a safe manner.
- Only undertake activities which you are trained and competent to carry out.
- Always behave in a way which does not put yourself or others at risk.
- Take reasonable care for yourself and others who may be affected.

and record the date. Part 1, 2 and the relevant sections in Part 3 should also be made known to non-employees, that is, visitors, temporary staff and contractors.

Monitoring, reviewing and revising the policy

Monitoring should be carried out at regular intervals, setting dates; so it is a planned process (Figure 17.1). Once the policy has been introduced into the practice you will need to assess if it is working for you, it is effective and doing what you intended it to do. Monitoring should include the following:

- Is everyone aware of the policy and do they understand its purpose?
- Are health and safety responsibilities allocated appropriately?
- Are people carrying out their work activities safely to an acceptable standard?

The review process is less frequent than monitoring and is intended to measure the overall success of the policy. Review must be planned in order to meet legal requirements (see section on legislation) and you should specify the period for review within an appropriate timescale, that is, every 12 months.

Reviews should address the following:

- Have there been any changes within the practice? For example:
  - □ Structural changes to the building
  - □ New personnel
  - □ Working arrangements and procedures
  - □ Introduction of new equipment
  - □ Developments in professional standards
  - □ Risk assessments identifying the need to improve working procedures

If these changes affect the practice from meeting its health and safety objectives then the policy must be revised. Revisions must be dated and brought to the attention of all employees and non-employees where relevant (Figure 17.1).

Summary

The content of your policy should be tailored to your individual practice and assist you in managing and developing your health and safety standards. It is a 'working document' that should reflect what is actually happening within your practice.

Action – check the following

- Are your working procedures carried out to an acceptable standard?
- Does your policy demonstrate the practice's commitment to the health and safety of everyone?
- Are roles and responsibilities clearly and accurately defined?
- Do your health and safety arrangements cover everything that you do?
- Is the policy communicated and distributed to everyone?
- Have you monitored the effectiveness of the policy?
- Have you reviewed your policy in the last 12 months?

Frequently asked questions

Q. The practice manager has signed our Health and Safety Policy; is this acceptable?

A. The most senior person, that is, the employer or practice owner, who has overall and ultimate responsibility for health and safety, must sign the policy as this demonstrates his/her commitment and control. Commitment and control must not be delegated to the practice manager.

Q. I am a single-handed practitioner. I only employ a nurse and receptionist; do I need a written Health and Safety Policy?

A. The law states that employers who employ less than five people at any one time are exempt from the requirement to have a **written** Health and Safety Policy; therefore, you do not need to state your policy in writing. However, you still need to demonstrate that you are committed to ensuring the health, safety and welfare of all those who may be affected by your activities.

Q. We currently have builders working in our premises. Why do they need to know about our Health and Safety Policy?

A. Both you and the contractor have duties under Health and Safety Law to protect each other and anyone else who might be affected by the work being undertaken. You need to know the risks involved in the work being carried out and how these will be controlled.

Similarly, the contractor must adhere to your working arrangements and cooperate to ensure the contract is managed safely.

Links to other chapters

Chapter 3 – Communication and training
Chapter 12 – Managing health and safety

In addition to the 'Links to other chapters' as stated above all the arrangements as stated in Part 3 of the policy are covered in this manual.

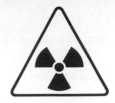

18 Radiation protection

Scope of this chapter

- Introduction – principles of radiation protection
- Legislation
- Ionising radiation safety
- Quality assurance and risk control
- Employees' responsibilities
- Cone beam computed tomography (CBCT)
- Radon gas
- Lasers (non-ionising radiation)
- Advice and information

Figures

Figure 18.1 – Radiation staff register.

Introduction – principles of radiation protection

The information provided in this chapter is designed to supplement and support the *Radiation Protection Quality Assurance Manual* used in all dental practices. This chapter is not intended to replace the manual and therefore at all times you should refer to and adhere to the quality assurance process as set out in the manual.

Although the risks associated with dental radiography are small in comparison to medical radiography, there remains a legal requirement to minimise the risk as far as is reasonably practicable. The principles of radiation protection can be classified into three categories; principles of justification, principles of optimisation and principles of limitation.

- Justification
  - The need for the use of radiation must be clearly identified prior to use.
  - The benefits of the use of radiation must outweigh the risks involved.
- Optimisation
  - The as low as reasonably achievable/practicable (ALARA/P) principle should be applied, keeping the dose of radiation used as low as is commensurate with a usable image.
- Limitation
  - The exposure of employees and patients should not exceed dose limits.
  - The need for retakes should be kept to an absolute minimum.
  - Safe practices should be adopted for staff involved with radiation procedures.

Legislation

- Ionising Radiation Regulations 1999 (IRR 1999):

  Every radiation employer shall, in relation to any work with ionising radiation that he undertakes, take all necessary steps to restrict so far as is reasonably practicable the extent to which employees and other persons are exposed to ionising radiation.

- Ionising Radiation (Medical Exposure) Regulations 2000 (IRMER 2000):

  The Regulations impose duties on those responsible for administering ionising radiation to protect persons undergoing medical exposure whether as part of their own medical diagnosis or treatment or as part of occupational health surveillance, health screening, voluntary participation in research or medico-legal procedures.

- The Management of Health and Safety at Work Regulations 1999:

  Employers [are] to make suitable and sufficient assessments of risks to health and safety of employees to identify the measures needed to remove the risks or reduce to an acceptable level.

Ionising radiation safety

- Authorisation must be granted by the Health and Safety Executive (HSE) for an employer to use electrical equipment intended to produce X-rays for the purpose of the exposure of patients for medical treatment.
- Notification of such use, or change of use, should be made in writing and contain the following information:
  - The name and address of the employer and a contact telephone or fax number or electronic mail address
  - The address of the premises where or from where the work activity is to be carried out and a telephone or fax number or electronic mail address at such premises
  - The nature of the business of the employer
  - That the source of the radiation is an electrical equipment
  - Whether any source is to be used at premises other than the address given above
  - Dates of notification and commencement of the work activity

A form, IRR3 Notification of Intention to Carry Out Site-Radiography – Ionising Radiation Regulations 1999 (Regulation 6(3), can be completed and sent to HSE Phoenix House, 23-25 Cantelupe Road, East Grinstead, West Sussex, RH19 3BE).

Notification must be received by HSE at least 7 working days in advance of commencement of work.

- Prior (proactive) risk assessment must be done when new X-ray equipment is planned, existing equipment is modified and when equipment is relocated.
- A suitable and sufficient assessment of the risk to any employee and other person must be carried out.
- Employers must adhere to dose limitations for women who are expecting or breastfeeding. Doses must not exceed 1 mSv to reduce the risk of bodily contamination. Employers should strongly encourage their staff to inform them as soon as pregnancy is confirmed by a medical practitioner. Women must be informed of the risks and control measures applied. Risk assessments should be reviewed and revised if necessary according to individual needs.
- Following annual dose limitations must not be exceeded *(IRR99)*:
  - Employees over 18 years — 20 mSV
  - Trainees aged under 18 — 6 mSv
  - Persons under the age of 16 — 1 mSv

Exposure must be restricted, where, reasonably practicable, below these limits.

- Contingency plans must be in place to address foreseeable accidents arising from the use of X-ray equipment.
- Appointment of (in writing) and consultation with a radiation protection advisor (RPA)

should take place to ensure compliance with the regulations.

- Identify the need for and involvement of a medical physics expert (MPE) to advise on patient doses (the MPE may also act as the RPA).
- Appoint one or more radiation protection supervisors (RPSs) to assist with compliance; this can be a dentist or dental nurse. The appointee must be competent to supervise the arrangements set out in local rules. Responsibilities may include the following:
  □ Providing support to staff on matters relating to radiation safety
  □ Maintaining the radiation staff register (Figure 18.1)
  □ Ensuring risk assessments are valid, current, suitable and sufficient in detail
  □ Assessing and identifying training needs
  □ Managing dose meter monitoring procedures
  □ Ensuring X-ray equipment is functioning correctly
  □ Reporting any defects or areas for concern
  □ Ensuring quality assurance and radiation safety is being implemented at all times

Figure 18.1 Radiation staff register.

All persons signing this register are confirming agreement to and acceptance of the roles and responsibilities as stated. The individual is also agreeing to comply with organisational and legal requirements for all aspects of radiation protection in relation to his/her specific role.

Name	Role	Responsibilities	Date of initial training	Date of review training	Signed
Example: Susan Smith	*Operator*	*Process and store films*	*25/01/2010*	*25/01/2015*	*Sue Smith*

- Identify persons who are required to act as 'operators' to assist with practical aspects of radiation procedures. Responsibilities may include the following:
  - Positioning the film, patient and X-ray tube head
  - Setting and directing the exposure (press the button)
  - Processing and storing films
  - Exposing test objects
- Designate staff as 'classified persons' if they are required to enter the controlled area; however, this is unlikely to be required.
- Employees who are engaged in work with ionising radiation are given appropriate training in the field of radiation. Training should include
  - the risks to health created by exposure to ionising radiation;
  - the precautions which should be taken; the importance of complying with the medical, technical and administrative requirements of the regulations; and
  - updation every 5 years covering topics recommended by statutory bodies.
- Every employer shall designate as a controlled area any area where steps need to be taken to minimise the risks of exposure to ionising radiation.
- Every employer shall consider the environment where ionising radiation is being directed and install appropriate physical barriers – for example, lead-lined and double-bricked walls and position equipment to reduce the risk of exposure to all persons.
- Every employer shall make and set down in writing such local rules as are appropriate to the radiation risk and the nature of the operations undertaken in that area.
- No person shall carry out a medical exposure unless it has been justified by the practitioner as showing a sufficient net benefit.
- In relation to all medical exposures to which the regulations apply the practitioner and the operator shall ensure that doses arising from the exposure are kept ALARP, consistent with the intended purpose.
- The employer shall draw up, keep up to date and preserve at each radiological installation

an inventory of equipment at that installation and, when so requested, submit it to the appropriate authority. Information required includes
  - name of manufacturer;
  - model number;
  - serial number or other unique identifier;
  - year of manufacture; and
  - year of installation.
- No practitioner or operator shall carry out a medical exposure or any practical aspect without having been adequately trained. This requirement does not prevent a person from participating in practical aspects of the procedure as part of practical training if this is done under the supervision of a person who himself/herself is adequately trained.
- The employer shall keep and have available for inspection by the appropriate authority an up to date record of all staff who have a responsibility for ionising radiation, in particular, radiation practitioners and operators engaged by him/her to carry out medical exposures. All of the above must have clearly defined tasks and permitted duties written down using actual names (Figure 18.1).
- Dose measurement services should be provided where applicable – for example, where it is suspected that individuals may receive dose levels that exceed 6 mSV per year. However, employers should be reducing these doses as low as is reasonable.

Quality assurance and risk control

Quality assurance programmes in dental radiography are designed to ensure that the principles of ALARA/P are applied effectively and should be comprehensive and inexpensive. The procedure adopted in the workplace should

- be documented;
- be the responsibility of a named person;
- use preferred methods of producing radiographs – the use of film holders as routine practice;
- monitor image quality – a simple subjective grading system is recommended and should

form part of the continual improvement target setting process. For example,

☐ Grade 1 = Perfect; no errors (70% should be grade 1)
☐ Grade 2 = Some errors, but not affecting diagnosis (no more than 20% should be grade 2)
☐ Grade 3 = Severe errors; non-diagnosis image (no more than 10% should be grade 3)

Consistently poor image quality on films will need to be investigated and causes addressed.

■ Monitor patient dose – ensure X-ray equipment is compliant with industry standards; for example, it should have an open-ended cone and be tested and maintained regularly.
■ Monitor darkroom procedures – ensure records are kept relating to the control of film stock, chemical changeover and equipment maintenance. It is a requirement that test films are used routinely to measure the overall performance of the processing equipment and processes.
■ Film storage – should be stored according to manufacturer's instructions, away from the source of radiation, heat or chemical contamination. Orthopantomograms (OPGs) should be stored upright to prevent pressure and sagging in the middle and intraorals stored on the side as opposed to being kept upright.
■ Care of extra-oral cassettes – never leave cassettes open when not in use; dust may settle and intensifying screens may be contaminated. Clean intensifying screen regularly with solution recommended by manufacturer. Never scratch intensifying screens to remove any dirt. Store cassettes to avoid the risk of damage, that is, place on stable surfaces.
■ Identify training needs – any training needs identified should be addressed and records kept of training undertaken.
■ Form part of an audit cycle – review of all areas within the quality assurance programme to ensure that it is compliant with current standards is required annually. Audits should be carried out by the person with overall control for the quality assurance programme. An audit

should be undertaken by an independent auditor every 3 years.
■ The information contained within the quality assurance programme should be used to assist with the review of the radiation risk assessment.

Employees' responsibilities

The responsibilities of employees working with ionising radiation are as follows:

■ Understand your specific role; an operator is anyone who carries out any part of an ionising radiation task.
■ Should not knowingly expose themselves or others to ionising radiation to a greater extent than is required for the purposes of their work.
■ Should exercise reasonable care while carrying out their work.
■ Should notify the employer immediately if they believe they or another person has received an overexposure.

Responsibilities of employees not working with ionising radiation are as follows:

■ Have a responsibility for your own radiation safety, your colleagues and others entering the premises.
■ Be familiar with the quality assurance and risk control measures applied in the practice.
■ Do not undertake any task unless trained to do so; this includes processing and storing films and radiographs.

Cone beam computed tomography (CBCT)

CBCT is designed for imaging a three-dimensional view of the patient's maxillofacial skeleton. It is particularly useful to undertake a radiographic assessment where the patient is suspected of having maxillofacial disease, for orthodontic, endodontic and periodontal treatment and for the placement of implants. It is relatively new in dental practices and there is much discussion about the safe use of the equipment in terms of radiation protection. The greatest importance is placed on the following *(Source: The Radiation Protection Implications of the Use of Cone Beam Computed Tomography (CBCT) in Dentistry – What You Need To Know J R Holroyd and A D Gulson.)*:

- The selection of equipment
- Establishment of a quality assurance programme
- Consultation with an RPA and an MPE
- Training requirements
- Dealing with referrals

The European Academy of Dental and Maxillofacial Radiology (EADMFR), who have a special interest in dental imaging of the maxillofacial region, recognised the need to set standards for the use of CBCT. In response to this need, EADMFR and the SEDENTEXCT project partners (individuals with an interest in radiation protection) collaborated to develop a set of 20 'basic principles' as follows *(Source: SEDENTEXT – Basic Principles for Use of Dental Cone Beam CT January 2009.)*:

1. CBCT examinations must not be carried out unless a history and clinical examination have been performed.
2. CBCT examinations must be justified for each patient to demonstrate that the benefits outweigh the risks.
3. CBCT examinations should potentially add new information to aid the patient's management.
4. CBCT should not be repeated 'routinely' on a patient without a new risk/benefit assessment having been performed.
5. When accepting referrals from other dentists for CBCT examinations, the referring dentist must supply sufficient clinical information (results of a history and examination) to allow the CBCT practitioner to perform the justification process.
6. CBCT should only be used when the question for which imaging is required cannot be answered adequately by lower dose conventional radiography.
7. CBCT images must undergo a thorough clinical evaluation ('radiological report') of the entire image dataset.
8. Where it is likely that evaluation of soft tissues will be required as part of the patient's radiological assessment, the appropriate imaging technique should be conventional medical computed tomography (CT) or magnetic resonance (MR), rather than CBCT.
9. CBCT equipment should offer a choice of volume sizes, and examination must use the smallest that is compatible with the clinical situation if this provides less radiation dose to the patient.
10. Where CBCT equipment offers a choice of resolution, the resolution compatible with adequate diagnosis and the lowest achievable dose should be used.
11. A quality assurance programme must be established and implemented for each CBCT facility, including equipment, techniques and quality control procedures.
12. Aids to accurate positioning (light beam markers) must always be used.
13. All new installations of CBCT equipment should undergo a critical examination and detailed acceptance tests before use to ensure that radiation protection for staff, members of the public and patient is optimal.
14. CBCT equipment should undergo regular routine tests to ensure that radiation protection, for both practice/facility users and patients, has not significantly deteriorated.
15. For staff protection from CBCT equipment, the guidelines detailed in Section 6 of the European Commission document *Radiation Protection 136 European Guidelines on Radiation Protection in Dental Radiology* should be followed.
16. All those involved with CBCT must have received adequate theoretical and practical training for the purpose of radiological practices and relevant competence in radiation protection.
17. Continuing education and training after qualification are required, particularly when

new CBCT equipment or techniques are adopted.

18. Dentists responsible for CBCT facilities who have not previously received adequate theoretical and practical training should undergo a period of theoretical and practical training that has been validated by a university or equivalent. Where national specialist qualifications in dentomaxillofacial radiology (DMFR) exist, the design and delivery of CBCT training programmes should involve a DMF radiologist.

19. For dentoalveolar CBCT images of the teeth, their supporting structures, the mandible and the maxilla up to the floor of the nose, clinical evaluation (radiological report) should be made by a specially trained DMF radiologist or, where this is impracticable, an adequately trained general dental practitioner.

20. For non-dentoalveolar small fields of view (e.g. temporal bone) and all craniofacial CBCT images (fields of view extending beyond the teeth, their supporting structures, the mandible, including the temporomandibular joint (TMJ) and the maxilla up to the floor of the nose), clinical evaluation should be made by a specially trained DMF radiologist or by a clinical radiologist (medical radiologist).

The above-mentioned principles are intended as an interim guidance and are correct at the time of writing (October 2009).

Radon gas

Definition

Like all sources of ionising radiation, radon gas is odourless, colourless and tasteless and, therefore, it is not easily detected. The gas being airborne, the primary route of exposure to humans is through inhalation and ingestion.

Risk factors

Radon is present in soil and can enter buildings by penetrating the foundations. In some areas, it is in the water if the water supply is from a well. Certain areas of the country pose a higher risk of radon than others, for example, Cornwall, Devon, Northamptonshire, parts of Derbyshire, Somerset and parts of the Grampian and Highland regions of Scotland. The construction of the building is important as radon can be drawn into the building through cracks in floors and gaps around pipes, cables and drains. High radon levels are uncommon above the ground floor of buildings but can be severe in lower ground levels, for example, cellars and basements. Radon levels are generally low in well-ventilated workplaces; however, problems have been found in more confined spaces such as shops and offices where ventilation is relatively low.

Testing for radon

It is the employer's duty to take action where it is suspected that radon is present above a defined level. The premises should be tested if the location, construction and ventilation make elevated radon levels seem likely and remedial work is carried out if required. A local HSE office or the local Council's Environmental Health Department provides advice on testing and remedial work.

Prevention

The risk to radon exposure can be reduced by improving or modifying ventilation systems, particularly in parts of the country which may be more at risk. Avoid the use of basements or cellars which are quite often used as waste storage areas in practices.

Lasers (non-ionising radiation)

Lasers are fast becoming the instrument of choice for dental procedures and safety is of paramount importance. Laser is an acronym for

- Light
- Amplification by
- Stimulated

- Emission of
- Radiation (meaning thermal radiation which is non-ionising).

Laser classes

Laser should conform to the British Standard BS EN 60825-1: 1994 incorporating Amendment Numbers 1, 2 and 3 September 2002; the revision is now referred to as *European Standard EN 60825-1*. Lasers are classified from group 1 (laser printers) to group 4. Dental equipment is usually classified as 3R, and 3B and 4 and must only be used under direct supervision of a trained and qualified dental or medical practitioner.

- Class 3R (IIIR) – this class replaces the former Class 3A, may have a maximum output power of 5 mW and have the potential to cause eye damage.
- Class 3B (IIIB) – may have an output power of up to 500 mW (half a watt) and could cause eye injury; the higher the output power the greater the risk of injury.
- Class 4 (IV) – has an output power of greater than 500 mW and there is no restriction on output power; this class has the capability to cause injury to eyes and skin and may also present a fire hazard.

Laser equipment must be labelled, indicating the specific classification.

Laser safety and quality assurance

- Practices wishing to provide laser treatment are required to apply for registration with the Care Quality Commission (CQC).
- The application involves checking, fitness of premises, fitness of persons and fitness of services and establishment.
- Practices will be inspected annually by CQC.
- Risk assessment and staff training are a mandatory requirement for practices using lasers.
- If you are considering new premises, CQC may send an inspector to check them for suitability, if you request it.

- Dental practitioners using Class 3B and Class 4 lasers must meet the minimum training requirements and gain informed consent from the patient.
- A laser protection advisor (LPA) must be appointed to advise on all aspects of laser safety (the LPA may also act as MPE).
- A laser safety officer (LSO) must also be appointed and be familiar with the manufacturer's safe operating procedures. Responsibilities include
  □ being familiar with all laser systems used in the practice;
  □ evaluating treatment areas;
  □ recommending and approving personal protective equipment/clothing (PPE/C) used;
  □ posting warning signs;
  □ implementing safe operating procedures;
  □ supervising the training of staff;
  □ equipment maintenance and calibration;
  □ significant event reporting and recording.

The LSO could be a dentist, hygienist or dental nurse and be trained to the required standard.

- Local rules are determined as are appropriate to the risk and the nature of the operations undertaken in that area and controlled zones established (as with ionising radiation).
- Appropriate warning signs are displayed in all areas where lasers are being used and unauthorised access prevented.
- Suitable and appropriate eye protection must be provided (according to manufacturer's instructions) and worn during all laser procedures. PPE must be cared for, stored and maintained to prevent damage and replaced when necessary.
- Laser equipment must be maintained according to the manufacturer's instructions.
- Primary Care Trusts (PCTs) may need to be informed of the use of laser equipment.

Advice and information

The National Radiological Protection Board (NRPB) merged with the Health Protection

Agency (HPA) on 1 April 2005 and resulted in a new division being formed to address radiation protection. The Radiation Protection Division of the HPA provides the following range of services:

- Research concentrating on the risks of radiation
- Identifying requirement of necessary protection
- Delivery of training
- Acting in an advisory role
- Providing the services of RPA, LPA and MPE

In addition to the above services the HPA provides the following information sources:

- Guidance Notes for Dental Practitioners on the safe use of X-ray equipment – National Radiological Protection Board – 2001
- Statutory Instrument 2000 No. 10.59 – The Ionising Radiation (Medical Exposure) Regulations 2000
- Statutory Instrument 1999 No. 3232 – The Ionising Radiations Regulations 1999
- Radiation protection (Quality Assurance Manual)
- European Academy of Dentomaxillofacial Radiology (EADMFR) – guidelines for the safe and ethical use of CBCT in dentistry
- The Medicines and Healthcare products Regulatory Agency (MHRA): Device Bulletin DB 2008(03) – *Guidance on the safe use of lasers, intense light source systems and LEDs in medical, surgical, dental and aesthetic practices*

Summary

Ionising radiation is a hazardous substance and its use is covered by two pieces of legislation. Employers must take all reasonable steps, as described throughout the chapter, to ensure that the risk of overexposure is minimised so far as is reasonably possible. Adequate training requirements should be identified for all members of the dental team involved in the practical aspects associated with radiographic examination. The use of lasers in dentistry must be carefully planned and executed. Lasers are capable of causing damage to the eyes, redness of the skin and breathing difficulties through inhalation of vapours. There is also a risk of fire and electric shock. Risks must be thoroughly assessed and suitable and appropriate control measures implemented to reduce the risk of harm to staff, the patient and anyone else who may be at risk.

Action – check the following

- Have you notified the HSE about your use of ionising radiation?
- Have you carried out ionising and non-ionising (if applicable) radiation risk assessments?
- Do you have adequate up to date records of equipment maintenance and staff training?
- Have you designated controlled areas and provided local rules?
- Do you need to consult with an RPA for any advice?
- Do you have a Quality Assurance Policy and Procedure related to radiation use?
- Does your Quality Assurance Procedure form part of your audit cycle?

Frequently asked questions

Q. Who needs personal dose measurement?

A. Those who are designated as 'classified persons' and therefore are likely to receive a dose exceeding 6 mSv per year should have arrangements in place where individual dose records are held. However, the primary aim of radiation protection is to reduce levels as low as is practicable.

Q. Who is a radiation protection advisor (RPA)?

A. The person or organisation that provides routine radiation surveys of the dental equipment would normally be expected to be able to act as RPA. The RPA consulted must be able to demonstrate compliance with the HSE's current criteria of competence for RPAs.

Q. What is the difference between a practitioner and an operator?

A. In terms of ionising radiation legislation 'practitioner' means a registered medical practitioner, dental practitioner or other health professional who is entitled in accordance with the employer's procedures to take responsibility for an individual medical exposure. An 'operator' means any person who is entitled, in accordance with the employer's procedures, to carry out practical aspects including those to whom practical aspects have been allocated.

Q. What should be in the local rules?

A. Local rule should include at least
- □ the name(s) of the appointed RPS(s);
- □ the identification and description of each controlled area and a summary of the arrangements for restricting access;
- □ an appropriate summary of the working instructions;
- □ identification or summary of any contingency arrangements indicating the reasonably foreseeable accidents to which they relate;
- □ the dose investigation level.

Q. What happens if a member of staff loses or damages his/her dosimeter?

A. The employer shall make an adequate investigation of the circumstances of the case with a view to estimating the dose received by that person during that period and either

(a) in a case where there is adequate information to estimate the dose received by that person, shall send to the approved dosimetry service an adequate summary of the information used to estimate that dose and shall arrange for the approved dosimetry service to enter the estimated dose in the dose record of that person; or

(b) in a case where there is inadequate information to estimate the dose received by the classified person, shall arrange for the approved dosimetry service to enter a notional dose in the dose record of that person which shall be the proportion of the total annual dose limit for the relevant period.

Q. What is non-ionising radiation?

A. Radiation which consists entirely of electromagnetic waves and does not release sufficient energy to ionise atoms.

Q. What adverse health effects can be caused by the use of lasers?

A. The retina and cornea of the eye can be affected by the output power of the wavelength. Lasers are capable of damaging the skin causing redness and burning. Inhalation of the vapours could cause nausea and breathing difficulties and in extreme cases the somatic cells are also susceptible to damage.

Links to other chapters

Chapter 7 – Electrical safety
Chapter 17 – Policy
Chapter 19 – Risk assessment
Chapter 22 – Work equipment

19 Risk assessment

Scope of this chapter

- Introduction
- Legislation
- Principles of risk assessment
- Types of risk assessment
- Risk assessment process
- Vulnerable groups

Figures

Introduction

Risk assessment is a vital tool to help you manage health and safety within your organisation. It is a proactive technique which should be undertaken before something goes wrong in order to determine what could cause harm to people. It will help you decide if you have taken sufficient precautions or whether more needs to be done in order to prevent accidents, which could result in injury or ill health. Risk assessments should form an integral part of your overall health and safety management system and be undertaken routinely, systematically and comprehensively. Risks to a person's health and safety exist in all workplaces, but a well thought out and appropriately applied risk assessment system will greatly help in managing these risks.

Legislation

The legal requirement to carry out risk assessment is categorised into three legislative groups:

- General – an Act of Parliament which places a broad requirement to reduce risks
- Specific – the legislation that categorically states that a risk assessment must be carried out for certain activities
- Implied – a risk assessment that may be required in order to determine if health and safety provisions are adequate and appropriate

Managing Health and Safety in the Dental Practice: A Practical Guide, by Jane Bonehill   © 2010 by Blackwell Publishing Ltd.

General

- Health and Safety at Work etc. Act 1974:

Employers must, so far as is reasonably practicable, control health and safety risks to which employees are exposed and others who might be affected by any of the organisations' undertakings.

Specific

- Management of Health and Safety at Work Regulations 1999:

*Every employer shall make a **suitable and sufficient** assessment of the risks to the health and safety of employees to which they are exposed and the risks of others who might be affected. A specific requirement exists to assess the risks to new and expectant mothers and women of reproductive age and young persons.*

- Health and Safety (Display Screen Equipment) Regulations 1992 (as amended):

Employers are required to make a suitable and sufficient assessment of the risks connected to workstations used by employees.

- Regulatory Reform (Fire Safety) Order 2005:

Employers must carry out a suitable and sufficient assessment of fire risks to which relevant people are exposed.

- Control of Substances Hazardous to Health Regulations 2002:

Employers are required to make a suitable and sufficient assessment of the risks to health caused by the use of hazardous substances.

- Manual Handling Operations Regulations 1992 (as amended):

Employers are required to make a suitable and sufficient assessment of the risks involved in manual handling operations where it is unreasonable to avoid the need for such activities.

- Ionising Radiation Regulations 1999:

Radiation employers must carry out a suitable and sufficient 'prior risk assessment' before commencing a new activity to which employees and others may be exposed.

Implied

- Personal Protective Equipment (PPE):

Employers to identify and provide suitable and appropriate PPE where risks can not be adequately controlled by other means.

- Health and Safety (First Aid) Regulations 1981:

Employers must have adequate and appropriate first aid equipment and facilities, however, the level of provision will depend on the risks present within the organisation.

Additional legal requirements

As identified above, there is a vast range of legislation that places a requirement on employers to undertake risk assessments. Employers must also be aware of additional requirements contained within the legislation and understand how to comply.

- A suitable and sufficient risk assessment
  - clearly identifies the risks presented and the level of severity;
  - provides detail in proportion to the risk;
  - considers everyone who may be exposed, both internal and external people;
  - states how long the risk assessment will remain valid and current;
  - identifies sources of advice for specialised risks.

In summary, the risk assessment must be suitable to the organisation and the activities undertaken and provide sufficient detail to demonstrate compliance.

- Recording risk assessment (Figures 19.1 and 19.2):
  - Where five or more are employed (includes self-employed), significant findings must be recorded.
  - Records must show that an adequate and accurate assessment was made.
  - There is an understanding of who might be affected.
  - All significant hazards were addressed and managed.
  - Reasonable precautions were taken to reduce the risk.

□ Residual risk levels are as low as is reasonable.

□ Employees should be involved in the process.

- Monitoring and reviewing risk assessments (Figure 19.3):

  □ Control measures are monitored for adequacy and appropriateness and remedial action taken where necessary.

□ Review is undertaken where it is suspected that the risk assessment is no longer valid or where changes occur.

Principles of risk assessment

Risk assessment is not just about controlling risks to ensure everyone is safe. It goes beyond

Figure 19.1 Situation-based risk assessment template.

Date:		RA NO:

LOCATION/WORK AREA:

ASSESSOR:	MANAGER:

Description of area/situation being assessed:

Hazards	People at risk	Risk factors
1.		
2.		
3.		
4.		
5.		
6.		

Risk rating						
Hazard effect (severity)			Likelihood			Overall risk
A	B	C	1	2	3	
1.						
2.						
3.						
4.						
5.						
6.						

(*continued overleaf*)

Figure 19.1   (*continued*)

Risk rating		Action priority
Hazard rate	**Risk rate**	**A1 –** Unacceptable, must receive immediate attention before work continues **A2/B1 –** Urgent, must receive attention as soon as possible to remove hazard or reduce risk **A3/C1 –** Must receive attention to reduce risk **B2 –** Should receive attention to reduce risk **B3/C2 –** Low priority, reduce risk after other priorities **C3 –** Very low priority, reduce risk after other priorities
A Death, major injury, major damage	**1.** Extremely likely to occur	
B Over 3-day injury, noteworthy damage	**2.** Probably likely to occur	
C Minor injury (first aid) Minor damage	**3.** Slight chance of occurring	

Current control measures (please list)

Current controls adequate?   Yes   No   (please circle)

Additional control required	Target date
1.	
2.	
3.	
4.	
5.	
6.	
7.	

Information, instruction or training needs

Monitoring (frequency)				Review (period)		
N/A	1 Month	3 Months	6 Months	3 Months	6 Months	12 Months

Who will monitor?	Who will review?
Method/s of monitoring	Method/s of review

Signatures	
ASSESSOR: JOB TITLE:	MANAGER:

Figure 19.2   Activity/task-based risk assessment template.

Date:		RA NO:

LOCATION/WORK AREA:	
ASSESSOR:	MANAGER:
Activity being assessed:	

Key tasks/method of work:

1.

2.

3.

4.

5.

6.

Hazards	People at risk	Risk factors
1.		
2.		
3.		
4.		
5.		
6.		

Risk rating						
Hazard effect (severity)			Likelihood			Overall risk
A	B	C	1	2	3	
1.						
2.						
3.						
4.						
5.						
6.						

Risk rating		Action priority
Hazard rate	**Risk rate**	**A1** – Unacceptable, must receive immediate attention before work continues
A Death, major injury, major damage	**1.** Extremely likely to occur	**A2/B1** – Urgent, must receive attention as soon as possible to remove hazard or reduce risk
B Over 3-day injury Damage to property/equipment	**2.** Frequent/often/likely to occur	**A3/C1** – Must receive attention to reduce risk **B2** – Should receive attention to reduce risk
C Minor injury, minor damage to property	**3.** Slight chance of occurring	**B3/C2** – Low priority, reduce risk after other priorities **C3** – Very low priority, reduce hazard or risk after other priorities

(*continued overleaf*)

Figure 19.2   (*continued*)

Current control measures (please list)

Current controls measures adequate? Yes No (please circle)	
Additional control required	**Target date**
1.	
2.	
3.	
4.	
5.	
6.	
7.	

Information, instruction or training needs	

Monitoring (frequency)				Review (period)		
N/A	1 Month	3 Months	6 Months	3 Months	6 Months	12 Months
Who will monitor?				Who will review?		
Method/s of monitoring				Method/s of review		

Signatures	
ASSESSOR:	MANAGER:
JOB TITLE:	

RA No	Date of assessment	Assessor	Additional controls Yes and date or No	Control measures monitoring date/s	Review date/s	Non-conformances (please state)	Signature and date

Figure 19.3 Risk assessment monitoring log.

this by providing a management system that demonstrates commitment to the organisation's Health and Safety Policy. It achieves this by the following means:

- Identifies hazards, assesses risks and implements controls
- Maintains an awareness of legal and ethical requirements
- Ensures competency of employees
- Demonstrates the communication of health and safety information
- Records significant findings and action taken to manage risks

Definitions

Before attempting to carry out risk assessments, it is important to have an understanding of the key terms used throughout the process.

- **Hazard** – something with the potential to cause harm; this can be split into two types of hazards: **safety** and **health** (Table 19.1).

It must be recognised that a hazard may fall into both categories. For example, when using a hazardous chemical, contact with the skin may cause a burn (safety) or if inhaled it could cause a respiratory condition (health). Leading on from the above two categories, hazards can then be grouped into five categories: biological, chemical, physical, ergonomic and organisational. Figure 19.4 provides examples of each category in relation to new and expectant mothers.

- **Risk** – the likelihood that the hazard is realised and the severity of harm.
- **Extent of risk** – calculated by determining several factors, for example, what is the risk, how the harm may be caused, the number of people affected and the severity of the consequences.
- **Control measures** – the arrangements made to reduce the risk as low as is reasonable.
- **Situation-based assessment** – assessment of an area or room where the hazard is static but could cause harm to people – for example, inadequate temperature or structural discrepancies (Figure 19.1).
- **Activity/task-based assessment** – breakdown of a main activity into component tasks, so hazards can be identified at each stage (Figure 19.2).

The benefits to the organisation of a properly designed and implemented risk assessment programme are as follows:

- It demonstrates compliance to legal requirements.
- It helps reduce accidents, injuries and ill health.
- It assists the organisation with improving performance standards.
- Staff feel cared for and therefore motivated to work as a team.
- The cost of injuries and ill health are reduced.
- Employers are at less of a risk of claims for compensation.
- It provides vital evidence to prove whether a duty of care has been breached.
- It helps in effective management of resources through a well-structured, planned approach which helps prioritise risks.
- It demonstrates good management practice.

Types of risk assessment

Your risk assessments should be specific to your organisation and clearly show what is present within your workplace that could put people at

Table 19.1　Types of hazards.

Safety	Health
Slips, trips and falls	Noise levels
Lifting and handling	Ionising radiation
Use of equipment	Biological agents
Fire	Hazardous chemicals
Electricity	Thermal environment
Sharp edges	Repetitive movement
Working alone	Poor lighting

Figure 19.4 New and expectant mothers' risk analysis.

In all cases consideration must be given to the unborn child, feeding infant and the new or expectant mother.

Hazards	Risk involved	Risk factors	Risk controls
Biological agents		Exposure may occur by	• Identify classification of biological agent female is exposed to Hazard Group (see Chapter 9)
Cytomegalovirus (CMV)	Transmission across placenta Close contact with children	• close contact with patients • inhalation or ingestion of exhaled respiratory secretions	• Obtain up to date patient medical history • Follow HTM 01-05 infection control procedures
Hepatitis B	Transmission through birth fluids	• inoculation from infected sharps, e.g. needles and decontamination procedures • contact with soiled materials, e.g. tissues or handkerchiefs	• Ensure immunisations are up to date • Review work activities, if necessary find alternative work
Hepatitis C	Transmission to unborn is rare		
Parvovirus Varicella zoster	Transmission across placenta	All activities that expose the person to the secretion of bodily fluids in particular, blood, saliva and vomit must be assessed	
Rubella HIV	Transmission across placenta and through breastfeeding		
Tuberculosis	Transmission via umbilical cord		
Chemical agents: Mercury Lead foil X-ray fluids Anaesthetic gases	Transmission through the placenta or breastfeeding may occur. Particular attention given to chemical agents with risk phrases: R40, R45, R46, R61, R63, R64 (see Chapter 9)	Exposure may occur by • inhalation of mercury vapours, ingestion or absorption through the skin; • inadvertent ingestion of lead dust (finger to mouth) • ingestion (finger to mouth) or inhalation of X-ray fluids • inhalation of nitrous oxide, halothane, isoflurane or enflurane	• Obtain risk phrase from MSDS (see Chapter 9) • Eliminate use of 'liquid mercury' or • Substitute 'liquid mercury' for capsules • Adequate ventilation in all areas • Provide gloves, masks and goggles (PPE) • Local (scavenger system) and general ventilation (open window) for GA/RA • Efficient hand hygiene • Health surveillance
Physical Ionising radiation	Significant exposure can be harmful to the fetus	Exposure may occur by • entering the IR controlled zone • taking high volumes of X-rays	• Ensure local rules are adhered to • Maintain at least 2-m exclusion zone • Limit number of X-rays taken
Extremes of heat	Heat tolerance is reduced Heat dehydration may impair breastfeeding	• inefficient ventilation causing heat stress • direct focus on light source may increase risk of headaches	• Provide adequate, adjustable ventilation • Provide tinted glasses when using light curing and enforce the use
Light curing units	Intolerance to extremes of light		

(continued overleaf)

Figure 19.4 *(continued)*

Hazards	Risk involved	Risk factors	Risk controls
Ergonomic Lifting and handling Prolonged sitting or standing Repetitive movement Confined work space	Miscarriage and premature birth After a caesarean section, lifting and handling is compromised Hormonal changes affecting ligaments increases risk of strain and sprain Excessive physical pressure on joints and swelling of the ankles As size increases dexterity, mobility and coordination may be reduced Breastfeeding mothers may be at greater risk from manual handling injuries *(Source: HSE)*	Exposure may occur by • moving and handling of stock • moving and handling of patients with impaired mobility or after anaesthesia • poorly organised work stations • receiving patients at reception while standing • treating patients while standing • inappropriate seating • inadequate workspace restricting movement	• Eliminate lifting and handling tasks • Alter the nature of the task • Allocate task to other staff • Adjust workstations to remove postural problems • Encourage staff to adjust working practices • Provide suitable adjustable seating and encourage staff to remain seated whilst working • Rearrange equipment and furniture to create more space
Organisational Stress Excessive workload Long hours Task responsibility Lone working	Excessive work pressure causing raised blood pressure	Exposure may occur by • long hours, back-to-back appointments, complex procedures and difficult patients • inability to react speedily and take flight where personal security is threatened • unable to summon immediate medical attention if unaccompanied	• Ensure hours and volume of work is not excessive • Longer or more frequent rest breaks, provide rest area • Organise and pace appointments efficiently, in particular complex treatments, i.e. implants/surgery • Eliminate lone working in later stages of pregnancy

risk. The risk assessment should be owned by you and show evidence that it is an analysis of your working environment and associated activities. Within the risk assessment framework, there are three main types of risk assessments.

- **Generic risk assessment**
  This type of assessment refers to general activities or common tasks that occur routinely throughout the practice. The activities or tasks are usually specific to a role, for example, dental nurse, and therefore could be undertaken by different people. It is important to identify any particular factors relating to the activity that may require a specific risk assessment to be undertaken.
- **Specific risk assessment**
  This type of assessment falls into two categories.
  1. A generic risk assessment may identify that particular factors exist which need to be further analysed and additional precautions taken. For example, the additional factors could be that the person carrying out the task might be inexperienced or is pregnant, the location where work is being undertaken is different or the equipment is different and therefore the risk presented differs from the original assessment.
  2. There may be instances where staff perform non-routine tasks or, non-standard functions take place which are not common to the normal day-to-day practice operations. Therefore, the task or function could pose a high degree of risk because of the unfamiliarity with the process and procedure and equipment involved – for example, any type of construction or maintenance work.
- **Dynamic risk assessment**
  This type of assessment is usually applied when staff are confronted with situations that could pose a risk to their personal safety. An example of this might be when dealing with conflict or with potentially violent individuals. A dynamic risk assessment requires individuals to continuously assess the situation as it unfolds in front of them and respond accordingly. A five-stage dynamic risk assessment model is represented below as **SATEN**.

1. Stop what you are doing; be aware of the situation and step back.
2. Assess the level of threat and analyse the environment, the person and any other factors that pose a risk.
3. Take action using the best option, make a reasonable excuse to leave the situation (flight) or deal with the situation (fight) and constantly monitor for changes.
4. Evaluate the success of the actions and determine if there is a need to incorporate the situation into the generic risk assessments.
5. Notify all those concerned or at risk and communicate the results of review of the generic risk assessments.

Individuals need a level of competence to be able to carry out a dynamic risk assessment and therefore you should identify those who will be most at risk from the situation.

Risk assessment process

Before implementing a risk assessment programme, the employer should appoint a competent person to assist with and coordinate the risk assessment process. Competencies required of an individual are as follows:

- Appreciate the aims and purpose of risk assessment.
- Have an understanding of legal requirements.
- Be aware of hazards that exist within the workplace.
- Understand the process for carrying out risk assessment.
- Be able to manage all stages of the risk assessment programme.
- Identify and allocate suitable resources.
- Know what to do with the results of the risk assessment.
- Appreciate the importance of being proactive in reporting and dealing with risks.
- Recognise own limitations and know when and where to seek further advice and assistance.
- Additional skills include communication, observational, analytical and problem-solving skills, time management and a systematic approach.

Figure 19.5   Hazard report form.

PERIOD FROM. . . . . :   **TO**. . . . .

Hazard identified	Location/work area	Identified by whom and date	Reported to whom and date
1.			
2.			
3.			
4.			
5.			
6.			
7.			
8.			
9.			
10.			
11.			
12.			
13.			
14.			
15.			

When this form is completed (15 hazards identified and reported), it should be placed in the health and safety management file.

The competent person may need to undertake specialised training in risk assessment to develop the above competencies. In addition to the competent person, everyone should be involved in the risk assessment programme. They should be encouraged to identify situations and conditions that are hazardous and, therefore, could cause harm and report them to the appropriate person for discussion so that action can be taken (Figure 19.5). Once you have appointed a competent person, the following process should be applied and written into your overall management system.

1. Plan the risk assessment programme

To ensure that your risk assessments consider all eventualities and demonstrate a commitment to your Health and Safety Policy, a well thought out and planned approach should be adopted.

The following should take place at the planning stage:

- Examine any previous risk assessment.
- Check existing safety policies and procedures and all associated documents.
- Decide the most suitable risk assessment template that covers all requirements.
- Decide the most suitable methods of hazard identification (see 2 below).
- Decide the risk rating formula and criteria to describe acceptable and unacceptable risks (see 4 below).
- Set health and safety objectives, inform and consult with your team.
- Decide on which activities/task-based assessments or situation-based assessments you are going to undertake.
- Decide how to break down work activities and areas and prioritise where to start.
- Obtain any relevant information from those working in the areas to be assessed.
- Agree with the team on what are classed as significant hazards.
- Determine whom to involve and at what stages.
- Consult with the team at planned stages throughout the process.
- Consider what training needs are required for those who will be directly involved.
- Consider what external sources of support, guidance or advice you may need.

2. Identify hazards

In the planning stage, you will have determined which risk assessment will be carried out on activities that are task based and those that are situation based. You will have decided which hazards are classed as significant and determined the most suitable and appropriate methods for identifying hazards from the list below:

- Walk tour inspections
- Feedback questionnaires from staff and patients (complaints)
- Observation of tasks being carried out
- On-job discussions
- Discussions and consultation during practice meetings

- Examination of accidents, ill health and absence records
- Personal experience
- Results of monitoring control measures or review of previous risk assessments
- Latest good practice or changes in legislation

Once the significant hazards have been identified you will then need to prioritise the order for assessment.

3. Identify who or what is at risk

Consider everyone who is likely to be exposed to the identified hazard including employees and non-employees and vulnerable groups (see below). In addition, the hazard may cause damage to property, equipment or materials.

4. Evaluate the risks

This stage can be quite complex as it requires an analysis of all **risk factors to determine how the hazard may present a risk**; risk factors include those associated with the following:

- Premises – for example, insufficient space or overcrowding
- Equipment and substances – for example, inadequate maintenance or improper use of substances
- Systems and procedures – for example, safe operating procedures not in place
- People not adhering to safety rules
- Organisational issues – for example, inadequate supervision
- Knowledge and skills of people – for example, training needs analysis not undertaken
- Design and layout – for example, no consideration given to equipment layout
- Management – for example, lack of understanding or commitment to health and safety

Evaluation also includes determining how serious the harm could be and the consequences, how frequently people are exposed to the hazard, the adequacy and suitability of existing controls, the likelihood of the harm being realised and the level of risk present and the overall risk rating. There

Table 19.2 Risk rating.

Hazard rate – severity and consequences	Risk rate – likelihood

A = Death
    Major injury
    Major damage
	1 = Extremely likely to occur

B = Off work for more than 3 days Noteworthy damage	2 = Probably likely to occur
C = Minor injury (first aid) Minor damage	3 = Slight chance of occurring
Overall risk rating	
A1 = Unacceptable; must receive immediate attention before work continues	
A2/B1 = Urgent; must receive attention as soon as possible to remove hazard or reduce risk	
A3/C1 = Must receive attention to reduce risk	
B2 = Should receive attention to reduce risk	
B3/C2 = Low priority; reduce risk after other priorities	
C3 = Very low priority; reduce risk after other priorities	

Source: Adapted from CIEH risk rating formula.

are several risk rating techniques that can be used and you will need to determine the most suitable. In dentistry, it is generally considered that a straightforward and simple qualitative rating is appropriate and you may find Table 19.2 useful.

5. Implement additional controls

Once you have determined the overall risk rating you need to decide on appropriate, suitable and reasonable control measures. You can either remove the hazard completely or reduce the level of risk to as low as is reasonably possible. In determining the most suitable control measures the hierarchy of controls should be applied. This is used in descending order where the first measure is the most effective and the last the least effective.

1. Eliminate or remove the hazard to avoid the risk.
2. Substitute the work activity for something less hazardous or risky.
3. Control the risk at source by separating or isolating people from the hazards.
4. Design safe working procedures appropriate to tasks and communicate to staff.
5. Ensure people have adequate supervision and receive appropriate information, instruction and training on job safety.
6. Provide personal protection in the form of equipment or clothing.
7. Provide other considerations, for example,
   □ health surveillance, for example, mercury screening;
   □ adequate and appropriate welfare facilities;
   □ first aid facilities;
   □ emergency procedures.

6. Record the risk assessment

As previously mentioned, there is a legal requirement to record the outcome of risk assessment where five or more people are employed. In addition to this, it is good management practice to make a record to facilitate communication, raise awareness and engage the whole team to encourage commitment. It also helps when you come to monitor the controls and carry out the overall review. It is useful to produce a record that summarises the risk assessments into a format that can be easily communicated to the team. An example of this summarised version can be found in Figure 19.3.

7. Monitor and review the risk assessment

Monitoring

Monitoring the control measures is a vital part of the risk assessment process. The purpose is to check that the controls that have been applied are working and reducing risk levels. This function should be allocated to the most appropriate people who will have access to and be directly involved in the activity or situation. It should be ongoing and frequent and controls should be maintained. Where there is reason to suspect controls are no longer appropriate, remedial action must be taken.

Review

Review of risk assessments is a less frequent process and should involve management. It should form part of the management system and be planned into the overall management strategy for the practice. The purpose is to identify if the risk assessment is still valid. Have significant changes occurred since the original assessment? Has there been an update in legislation or good practice or are unsafe working practices being undertaken? It is recommended that review takes place at least every 5 years.

Vulnerable groups

Certain classes of workers may be more vulnerable and therefore more at risk from hazards and risks because of their individual circumstances. Those listed here are considered in terms of the dental environment:

New and expectant mother

A new and expectant mother is one who (Figure 19.4)

- has given birth in the last 6 months, (given birth is defined as: 'delivered a living child or after 24 weeks of pregnancy, a stillborn child'); or
- is breastfeeding; there is no time limit on the period of breastfeeding; this is for the mother to decide;
- is pregnant.

Evidence suggests that women are working longer into their pregnancies and therefore, employers need to be more aware of workplace risks associated with pregnancy. Female employees must be encouraged to inform the employer in writing as soon as the pregnancy is confirmed by a medical practitioner. The requirement to inform the employer should be written into the practice Health and Safety Policy and also contained within the contract of employment. The following process should then be undertaken with the expectant mother:

- A review of the generic risk assessments is undertaken with the individual in order to identify any specific issues that may put her or the unborn child more at risk (specific risk assessment). Any medical advice received about the individual should also be taken into account as should the general effects of pregnancy on the body; for example:
  - □ Morning sickness
  - □ Changes in blood pressure
  - □ Backache
  - □ Varicose veins
  - □ Haemorrhoids
  - □ Fluid retention
  - □ Pressure on the bladder
  - □ Tiredness and fatigue
  - □ Headaches
  - □ Increase in size
  - □ Shortness of breath
  - □ Balance
  - □ Carpal tunnel syndrome
  - □ Emotional changes

- Suitable and adequate controls should then be determined and applied to her work activities to reduce risks.
- The controls should be monitored to ensure they remain suitable and risk assessments must be reviewed with the expectant mother at planned intervals. This should normally take place at each trimester, or if her condition changes or if there are significant changes to her work activity.
- If risks cannot be suitably and adequately controlled then the employer must alter hours of work or working conditions.
- If alterations are unreasonable or the risks would still remain, then suitable and alternative work must be found.
- If alternative work cannot be found then the employer must suspend the employee for as long as necessary with full pay (except where alternative work has been refused).
- Rest areas should be provided for expectant mothers where they can lie down.

Employers may need to seek advice from occupational health or medical practitioners on vaccine status during pregnancy or if there is a need for prophylactic vaccinations. Maternity rights allow the expectant mother time off from work with full pay for antenatal appointments. Remember everyone experiences pregnancy differently; however, it must be treated as a condition and not an illness.

Return to work

The mother's body will still be readjusting to both physical and emotional changes. This needs to be taken into consideration when the maternity period has come to an end and the new mother returns to work. The following adjustments should be made as follows:

- If the mother is breastfeeding, (she has the right to choose the period), before returning to work she should notify the employer in writing.
- When the new mother returns to work, a 'back to work' specific risk assessment should be undertaken and if necessary reasonable adjustments made to her work activities and environment.

- Rest areas should be provided for breastfeeding mothers.
- It is recommended that a private, safe and healthy area is provided for mothers to express milk and store it in a refrigerator.
(*Source: HSE*)

A young person

- A young person is defined as someone who is under 18 years of age.
- A child is defined as 'someone who is over 13 years of age but has not reached compulsory school leaving age'.

Young persons (and children) are more at risk because of their inexperience of work patterns and workplace demands and their psychological ability and immaturity. The following human factors should be considered when assessing the risks to both groups (without prejudice):

- Perception of risk
- Peer influence and values approved by peer group
- Parental influences and family attitudes
- Conflicts between what is factually right and what the young person believes to be right
- Gender characteristics, both physical and psychological
- Taking unacceptable risks because of the fear of non-achievement or willingness to please

The practice may have carried out a 'young person's' generic risk assessment. However, prior to the young person starting work, a specific risk assessment must be undertaken. This must involve the young person and the outcomes communicated to him/her. The extent of residual risk will determine what restrictions or prohibitions are placed on his/her work activities. In addition to the human factors listed above, the following should be considered when carrying out the specific risk assessment:

- Work that is beyond the person's physical or psychological ability
- Exposure to biological agents prior to immunisation status being confirmed

- Exposure to hazardous chemical agents where controls must be applied
- Directing the exposure for ionising radiation must be prohibited
- The type, range and use of hazardous work equipment, in particular pressure vessels
- Specific tasks that require complex safe operating procedures, for example, during implant procedures
- Any other factors that could put the individual at risk of being injured or suffer ill health

A young person must, at all times, be supervised by a competent person. He/she must know how to report concerns and not carry out tasks which he/she is unfamiliar with or has not been trained on.

Children

Certain requirements are placed on employers if they employ people under the minimum school-leaving age. Children who have reached 13 years of age but are under 15 years may be employed to do 'light work' for no more than 5 hours on any non-school day which is not a Sunday. Children of 15 years or more may be employed for no more than 8 hours on any non-school day. During school holidays, a limit of 25 working hours per week is placed on children under 15 years and a limit of 35 hours per week for children over 15 years. Children working for more than 4 hours must have a rest break of 1 hour. During school holidays two consecutive weeks must be kept free from employment *(Source: Croner's Health and Safety A-Z)*. The limits in respect of a 'child' described in this chapter are an absolute must and the child cannot decide to extend these limits. If the practice is providing 'work experience' (WE) for a 'child' as part of his/her vocational education and training programme, a risk assessment must be undertaken prior to the WE period and the parent or guardian informed of the outcome. If the outcome shows that risk levels are unacceptable and cannot be reasonably adjusted, the practice will need to decide if they can act as WE providers. This is usually managed and coordinated by the school or education establishment arranging the training.

Women of reproductive age

All 'reproductive hazards' associated with their work activities should be considered for women of child-bearing age – for example, work involving ionising radiation, general and relative anaesthesia and certain chemicals.

Lone workers

Hazards arising from conflict or violence and aggression should be considered as should procedures for dealing with an emergency situation.

Disabled workers

Access and egress to and from the workplace may be more difficult, particularly in emergency situations. Physical and sensory impairment must be considered when using work equipment or communicating health and safety information.

Temporary/Locum staff

The temporary staff may be more at risk because they are unfamiliar with the practice's specific systems, policies and procedures and the working environment.

Work returnees

Significant changes may have occurred and adapting and adjusting takes time. For some, the transition period could be difficult and therefore more time may be needed to readjust, and increased levels of supervision may be needed.

Visitors and contractors

Visitors and contractors will be unfamiliar with the workplace and therefore unaware of the hazards present. In addition, they may inadvertently create a hazard without realising the risks associated or who might be affected.

Task

From the above list identify those people who may be more at risk in your practice and therefore classed as vulnerable groups. Make a suitable and sufficient assessment and implement the necessary controls.

Summary

Risk assessments assist in proactively managing health and safety. The aim of risk assessments is to improve standards and reduce the risk of injury, ill health and damages. Everyone should take responsibility for identifying hazards and risks associated with his/her own job role and determining suitable and sufficient means of control.

Action – check the following

- If you are carrying out risk assessments, have you been trained and are you competent in the process?
- Do your practice risk assessments actually identify what hazard and risks are present in your own organisation and how you have suitably and adequately controlled the risks?
- Do your risk assessments identify those especially at risk who may be classed as 'vulnerable groups'?
- Are your risk assessments up to date, have they been reviewed recently and revised if necessary?

Frequently asked questions

Q. We have purchased risk assessments from a reputable source; can we use these as evidence to demonstrate that we have carried out the process?

A. The Management of Health and Safety at Work Regulations requires employers (or nominated person) to carry out a suitable and sufficient assessment of risks present within their working environment. Therefore, risk assessments purchased from elsewhere may not meet this requirement unless the assessor has physically spent time in your practice and undertaken the process as described in this chapter. Your employees are the best people to take part in the risk assessment process as they will have first-hand knowledge and experience of the day-to-day operations, what hazards may exist and how they present a risk. Risk assessments that you have purchased could be used as guidance to help you carry out and coordinate your risk assessment programme.

Q. What is the difference between monitoring and reviewing in the risk assessment process?

A. Monitoring generally relates to frequently checking that the control measures applied are still in place, being adhered to and used correctly and are reducing the risk as intended. Review is less frequent and should be part of the overall management process; its purpose is to ensure that risk assessments remain valid.

Q. When should risk assessments be reviewed?

A. There is no time period stated in law for risk assessments to be reviewed; however, it is recommended that this should take place when changes occur which could make the previous assessment invalid – for example, if an activity changes or a new piece of equipment is purchased. It is good practice to build a planned review into your overall management audit system as this will demonstrate that your risk assessments remain up to date, and are reliable and valid.

Links to other chapters

Chapter 1 – Accidents and first aid
Chapter 4 – Conflict management
Chapter 6 – Display screen equipment
Chapter 8 – Fire safety and emergencies
Chapter 9 – Hazardous substances
Chapter 11 – Lone working
Chapter 12 – Managing health and safety
Chapter 13 – Manual handling
Chapter 16 – Personal protective equipment
Chapter 18 – Radiation protection

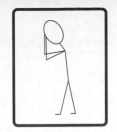

20 Stress management

Scope of this chapter

- Introduction
- Legislation
- Definition
- Effects of stress
- Recognising stress – signs and symptoms
- Workplace stressors
- Preventing and managing work-related stress

Figures

Introduction

Stress is now recognised as a significant workplace hazard. Recent figures from the Health and Safety Executive (HSE) show that around 500,000 people a year claim illness from work-related stress. This shows that stress is a major issue that employers need to address. Factors that have the potential to cause stress exist in all dental environments. If these factors are not identified and managed, they will have a serious effect on a person's physical and psychological health and well-being. This in turn will be detrimental to the efficiency and operation of the business. Organisations should take a proactive approach to preventing stress and demonstrate a duty of care to the employees.

Legislation

- Health and Safety at Work etc. Act 1974:

  Employers have a general duty to ensure, so far as is reasonably possible, the health, safety and welfare of all employees. The general duty covers the physical and psychological well-being of employees and the individual needs of each employee should be considered.

- Management of Health and Safety at Work Regulations 1999:

  Employers [are] to make suitable and sufficient assessments of risks to health and safety of employees to identify the measures needed to remove the risks or reduce to an acceptable level. This includes ensuring employees have the physical and psychological capabilities to carry out tasks.

Managing Health and Safety in the Dental Practice: A Practical Guide, by Jane Bonehill   © 2010 by Blackwell Publishing Ltd.

- Working Time Regulations 1998 (as amended):

    Excessive working hours are a contributory factor to work related stress. Employers must limit the amount of hours an employee works to 48 hours a week averaged over a 17 week period. In work, daily and weekly rest breaks must be provided and employers will need to keep a record if employees decide to opt out of the Regulations.

Definition

A range of definitions of stress exist. This is mainly due to different opinions, individual responses to stress, people's experiences and, for some, the reluctance to identify that stress is a problem. Some of the more common definitions are as follows:

- 'Stress is a condition or feeling experienced when a person perceives that demands exceed the personal and social resources the individual is able to mobilise' (*Richard S. Lazarus*).
- 'A force acting on or within someone and acting to distort it' (*Oxford dictionary*).
- 'Interference that disturbs a person's healthy mental and physical well-being' (*D&K Essential Managers Guide*).
- 'An adverse reaction that people have to excessive pressure or other types of demands placed upon them' (*Health and Safety Executive*).

The above shows that there is no single definition of stress and that stress does not indicate personal faults or weaknesses. Stress is about negative experiences that need to be managed. It should be recognised that most of us work under a certain amount of pressure, but it is when the pressure becomes unreasonable and destructive that there is a problem.

Effects of stress

Work-related stress does not just affect the health and well-being of an individual. It has a knock-on effect on their families and friends and ultimately will have an impact on the business. These effects may be both short and long term. If stress is identified early enough, long-term effects could be greatly reduced. It must also be recognised that individuals suffering from stress may be at a greater risk of having an accident.

Effects on an individual

Stress is personal to an individual. Everyone copes with situations and problems differently and the individual's genetic make-up also affects the way he/she handles life. However, employers need to have an understanding of the more general effects of stress such as the following:

- Physical health
    - High blood pressure and raised metabolic rate
- Mental health
    - Anxiety attacks, mood swings and behavioural changes
- Decision-making
    - Rational thinking is diminished, lose sight of aims and goals

Effects on families and friends

- The individual may be unable to leave work-related problems at work. Family issues that are normally easily resolved escalate. This may lead to a change in family circumstances and could result in loss of income, further adding to the stress.
- The individual may withdraw from normal social activities and destroy social relationships.

Effects on the business

- Quality of service – the well-being of an individual can affect the way he/she deals with customers/patients. If the quality of service is reduced, there may be an increase in complaints and customers/patients could go elsewhere.

- Reputation – dissatisfied customers/patients may tell others of the poor service they received.
- Morale of staff – motivation levels will be low and disputes could happen between colleagues, resulting in mistrust.
- Staff retention – people may be absent because of sickness and employees could leave. Recruitment and selection to replace staff is a cost to the business.

Recognising stress – signs and symptoms

The approach to stress throughout this chapter is for employers to be proactive so that they can identify how stress may be caused, with the aim being prevention. In order to do this effectively, employers need to be able to recognise the signs and symptoms individuals may be experiencing and encourage them to report to occupational health, human resources or their managers so that it can be discussed and addressed immediately. Signs and symptoms of stress are grouped as follows:

Physical

- Chest pain and palpitations
- High blood pressure
- Breathlessness
- Nausea
- Aches and pains
- Headaches
- Digestive disorders
- Sleep problems/tiredness
- Slouched posture
- Profuse sweating
- Bloodshot eyes
- Dishevelled clothing

Emotional

- Mood swings
- Feeling anxious
- Feeling depressed
- Loss of sense of humour
- Becoming more cynical
- Loss of enthusiasm
- Aggressiveness
- Poor concentration
- Decrease in confidence and self-esteem
- Being tearful

Behavioural

- Drop in work performance
- Excessive drinking and smoking
- Drug abuse
- Overeating/loss of appetite
- Change in sleep patterns
- Poor time management
- Obsessive or erratic behaviour
- Poor judgement
- Overreacting to situations
- Indecisiveness and forgetfulness

Psychological (negative thoughts)

- 'I am a failure'.
- 'I should be able to cope'.
- 'I can't cope'.
- 'No one understands'.
- 'Why am I being picked on?'
- 'What's the point in doing this?'
- 'I can't remember where I put it'.

External factors should also be recognised. For example, a staff member may be experiencing personal problems which could be affecting the way he/she performs at work.

Workplace stressors

In November 2004, the HSE developed *The Management Standards for Work-related Stress* in order to reduce the levels of stress. The standards cover seven key areas of work. The list below addresses the primary causes of stress in relation to the seven key areas. The Workplace Stressors Staff Risk Assessment (Figure 20.1) is a

Figure 20.1   Workplace stressors staff risk assessment.

The following statements have been adapted from the Health and Safety Executive's (HSE's) *Management Standards for Work-Related Stress*. This risk assessment will help you to identify what in your organisation may be causing you stress and enable action to be taken. All responses should be treated in strictest confidence and used only for the intended purpose. Respond to each statement by placing a ✓ in the relevant column.

DATE:				
Standard	**Statement**	**Always**	**Sometimes**	**Never**
1. Culture	1.1 The practice identifies the causes of stress			
	1.2 I am encouraged to report to my manager if I feel under pressure			
	1.3 I receive support and my concerns are acted upon			
	1.4 Morale is high and positive within our organisation			
2. Demands	2.1 I am clear on what is expected of me at work			
	2.2 My capabilities to do my job are assessed			
	2.3 I have achievable targets			
	2.4 If work gets difficult my colleagues help me			
	2.5 My concerns are addressed and acted upon			
3. Control	3.1 I have a say in my own pace of work			
	3.2 I am involved in decision-making			
	3.3 I am encouraged to progress and develop			
	3.4 We have an open communication process			
	3.5 I am consulted on about my work pattern			
4. Support	4.1 I receive support from my colleagues			
	4.2 My manager will assist me with a problem			
	4.3 My manager encourages me to progress			
	4.4 I am given supportive feedback on my work			
	4.5 I know who I directly report to			
5. Relationships	5.1 I can talk to my manager if a colleague has treated my unfairly			
	5.2 My manager promotes fairness and equality			
	5.3 My manager deals with unacceptable behaviour fairly			
	5.4 I feel we have a positive approach to team working			
6. Role	6.1 I am clear about my role and responsibilities			
	6.2 The activities I perform are compatible with my level of competence			

Figure 20.1 *(continued)*

Standard	Statement	Always	Sometimes	Never
	6.3 I understand my position within the organisation			
	6.4 I am able to discuss any concerns about my role and responsibilities			
	6.5 I receive training to ensure that my competence remains valid and current			
7. Change	7.1 I am informed about any changes before they happen			
	7.2 I am given the opportunity to discuss changes			
	7.3 I am encouraged to put my point of view across about impending changes			
	7.4 I am supported by my manager during the change process			
	7.5 I receive training to assist with managing change			
From your responses please list below the three priority areas that have the potential to cause you stress; these should be discussed with your manager to determine an appropriate course of action.				
1.				
2.				
3.				

useful aide-mémoir to help identify development areas.

- **Culture** – an organisation where stress is regarded as an acceptable part of the job is therefore the norm and people are expected to cope, and performance is the priority.
- **Demands** – excessive and unreasonable demands; workloads are heavy or people are bored (underemployed); resources are minimal; quantity is a priority over quality.
- **Control** – people have no say in the way they work; communication is not encouraged and consultation is non-existent.
- **Support** – an autocratic boss/manager; a blame culture exists; little encouragement to progress; lack of supervision. Training is seen as an expensive and unnecessary resource.

- **Relationships** – bullying and harassment, rumours and gossip is the norm; unacceptable behaviour is not addressed. There is negative interaction between employees.
- **Role** – no clear guidance or job descriptions; people unsure of their status or responsibilities; tasks are split between colleagues and training is lacking.
- **Change** – change in job role and adjusting to new situations; being downgraded, relocation, new technology, uncertainty about the future of the organisation.

In this section, we have applied the HSE's Management Standards to help identify the causes of stress. In the next section, we will use the standards to help prevent and manage work-related stress.

Preventing and managing work-related stress

Organisations should start by designing and implementing a Stress Management Policy that clearly expresses the employer's commitment to tackling stress. Commitment should be expressed as follows:

- Job design minimises stress factors.
- Working environment is suitable and fit for the purpose.
- Management actively takes a positive approach to prevent or reduce the risk.
- Provide support for those who are suffering from stress.

The policy should define stress and clearly state the responsibilities of individuals. Roles and responsibilities could be expressed as in the following section.

Roles and responsibilities

- Employer:
  - Design a stress management policy aimed at prevention.
  - Provide necessary resources including training and counselling.
  - Assess workplace risks and implement control measures to eliminate or reduce the causes to prevent individuals from becoming ill.
- Manager:
  - Implement the policy.
  - Be aware of what could cause stress and identify the signs.
  - Monitor work loads.
  - Implement risk control measures and monitor effectiveness.
  - Identify specific training needs to assess capabilities.
  - Ensure that effective communication processes exist.
  - Encourage staff to report concerns and support them in resolving these.

- Seek support from other agencies where necessary.
- Occupational health:
  - Provide specialist advice.
  - Train and support managers and employers.
  - Support individuals through the term of any illness and provide a return-to-work programme where necessary.
  - Keep employer informed of any legal and professional changes in the approaches to stress management.
- Employees:
  - Identify causes and report concerns to management.
  - Work with your employer and manager to reduce the risk of stress.
  - If stress is experienced, the employee should talk to someone about how they feel. This could be an independent person, who may be able to provide appropriate advice and help. This could be the individual's general practitioner (GP) or a trained counsellor.

Finally, the policy should state the arrangements in place to proactively manage stress. The arrangements will be determined through a suitable and sufficient risk assessment which is aimed at meeting the requirements of the HSE's Management Standards. Consultation should take place between employer, manager and employees to ensure that the policy meets organisational and individual requirements.

A stress management risk assessment should incorporate the following:

- **Step 1 – identify the hazards**
  - Analysis of tasks and methods of working. Gather existing data on sickness/absence, accidents and staff turnover due to stress and carry out staff surveys on attitudes and relationships, organisational culture and general morale.
- **Step 2 – identify who might be at risk and how**
  - Establish who is most at risk and acknowledge that stress can affect anyone. Identify those who may be more vulnerable than others, for example, previous sufferers.

Consider how people may be affected and the groups who are most at risk.

- **Step 3 – evaluate the risk**
  - □ Determine the impact and the severity of the situation if stress is not addressed and identify priority areas to reduce the risk of stress.
- **Step 4 – implement control measures**
  - □ Evaluate options to control stress and develop an action plan for implementation of the control measures. Document the findings and outcomes.
- **Step 5 – monitor and review**
  - □ Measure the impact of actions taken, identify any new risks and amend existing controls and ensure continuous improvement.

Applying the HSE's Management Standards

Adapted from HSE's *Tackling Stress: The Management Standards Approach*.

The Organisation Staff Management Standards questionnaire (Figure 20.2) can help you to assess how well you are meeting the stress management criteria.

The following describes the HSE's approach to managing stress in the workplace; it sets out the standards expected of the organisation. The organisation questionnaire (Figure 20.2) should be used to assess if the required standard is being achieved and will help the employer to identify development areas.

- **Culture – organisational approach and recognition of causative factors:** The standard is that
  - □ the organisation recognises that stress is a health and safety issue and is positive and proactive in its approach to controlling it;
  - □ it will have good communications and provide support at all levels.
- **Demands – workload, work patterns and the work environment:** The standard is that
  - □ employees indicate that they are able to cope with the demands of their jobs;

  - □ Systems are in place to respond to any individual concerns.
- **Control – how much say the person has in the way he/she does his/her work:** The standard is that
  - □ employees indicate that they are able to have a say about the way they do their work;
  - □ systems are in place to respond to any individual concerns.
- **Support – includes the encouragement, assistance and resources provided by the organisation, management and colleagues:** The standard is that
  - □ employees indicate that they received adequate information and support from their colleagues and superiors;
  - □ systems are in place to respond to any individual concerns.
- **Relationships – includes promoting positive working to avoid conflict and dealing with unacceptable behaviour:** The standard is that
  - □ employees indicate that they are not subjected to unacceptable behaviours;
  - □ systems are in place to respond to any individual concerns.
- **Role – whether people understand their role within the organisation and whether the organisation ensures that the person does not have conflicting roles:** The standard is that
  - □ employees indicate that they understand their role and responsibilities;
  - □ systems are in place to respond to any individual concerns.
- **Change – how organisational change is managed and communicated in the organisation:** The standard is that
  - □ employees indicate that the organisation engages them frequently when undergoing an organisational change;
  - □ systems are in place to respond to any individual concerns.

Measuring performance

Once the control measures and management standards have been implemented there will be a need to monitor the effectiveness to ensure that

Figure 20.2   Organisation stress management standards.

The template has been adapted from the Health and Safety Executive's (HSE's) *Management Standards for Work-Related Stress*. The standard sets out the criteria and the statement describes what the organisation should aim to achieve in order to demonstrate a commitment to preventing work-related stress. It will help to identify what is already in place (how demonstrated) and if 'action' is required to meet the standard. It should be used together with Workplace Stressors Staff Risk Assessment.

1. Culture	**Standard:** Organisational approach and recognition of causative factors • The organisation recognises that stress is a health and safety issue, and is positive and proactive in its approach to controlling it • The organisation has good communications and provide support at all levels		
	Statement – aim to achieve	**How demonstrated**	**Action**
	1.1 The organisation is committed to preventing and managing stress		
	1.2 Staff are encouraged to report to management if they feel under pressure		
	1.3 Management provides support and concerns are acted upon		
	1.4 Morale is high and positive within the organisation		
2. Demands	**Standard:** Workload, work patterns and the working environment • Employees indicate that they are able to cope with the demands of their jobs • Systems are in place to respond to any individual concerns		
	Statement – aim to achieve	**How demonstrated**	**Action**
	2.1 Employees are provided with adequate and achievable demands in relation to the agreed hours of work		
	2.2 People's skills and abilities are matched to the job demands		
	2.3 Tasks are designed to be within the capabilities of employees		
	2.4 Employees' concerns about their work environment are addressed and acted on		
3. Control	**Standard:** Workload, work patterns and the working environment • Employees indicate that they are able to cope with the demands of their jobs • Systems are in place to respond to any individual concerns		
	Statement – aim to achieve	**How demonstrated**	**Action**
	3.1 Where possible, employees have control over their pace of work		
	3.2 Employees are encouraged to use their skills and initiative to do their work		
	3.3 Where possible, employees are encouraged to develop new skills to help them undertake new and challenging work		
	3.4 Employees are encouraged to communicate work-related issues		
	3.5 Employees are consulted over their work patterns		

Figure 20.2 *(continued)*

4. Support	**Standard:** Encouragement, assistance and resources provided by the organisation, management and colleagues • Employees indicate that they receive adequate information and support from their colleagues and superiors • Systems are in place to respond to any individual concerns		
	Statement – aim to achieve	**How demonstrated**	**Action**
	4.1 The organisation has policies and procedures which adequately support employees		
	4.2 Systems are in place to enable and encourage managers to support their staff		
	4.3 Systems are in place to enable and encourage employees to support their colleagues		
	4.4 Employees know what support is available and how to access it		
	4.5 Employees know how to access the required resources to do their job		
	4.6 Employees receive regular and constructive feedback		
5. Relationships	**Standard:** Promote positive working to avoid conflict and deal with unacceptable behaviour • Employees indicate that they are not subjected to unacceptable behaviours • Systems are in place to respond to any individual concerns		
	Statement – aim to achieve	**How demonstrated**	**Action**
	5.1 The organisation promotes positive behaviours to avoid conflict and ensure fairness		
	5.2 Employees share information relevant to their work		
	5.3 The organisation has agreed policies and procedures to prevent or resolve unacceptable behaviour		
	5.4 Systems are in place to enable and encourage managers to deal with unacceptable behaviour		
	5.5 Systems are in place to enable and encourage employees to report unacceptable behaviour		
6. Role	**Standard:** Whether people understand their role within the organisation and whether the organisation ensures that the person does not have conflicting roles • Employees indicate that they understand their role and responsibilities • Systems are in place to respond to any individual concerns		
	Statement – aim to achieve	**How demonstrated**	**Action**
	6.1 The organisation ensures that, as far as possible, the different requirements it places upon employees are compatible		

(continued overleaf)

Figure 20.2   (*continued*)

	6.2 The organisation provides information to enable employees to understand their role and responsibilities		
	6.3 The organisation ensures that, as far as possible, the requirements it places upon employees are clear		
	6.4 Systems are in place to enable employees to raise concerns about any uncertainties or conflicts they have in their roles and responsibilities		
7. Change	**Standard:** How change is managed and communicated in the organisation • Employees indicate that the organisation engages them frequently when undergoing an organisational change • Systems are in place to respond to any individual concerns		
	Statement – aim to achieve	**How demonstrated**	**Action**
	7.1 The organisation provides employees with timely information to enable them to understand the reasons for proposed changes		
	7.2 The organisation ensures adequate employee consultation on changes and provides opportunities for employees to influence proposals		
	7.3 Employees are aware of the probable impact of any changes to their jobs. If necessary, employees are given training to support any changes		
	7.4 Employees are aware of timetables for change		
	7.5 Employees have access to relevant support during changes		

If you have identified action is required by the organisation in order to meet the Management Standards please state below what the organisation needs to do in the relevant sections.

1. CULTURE:

2. DEMANDS:

3. CONTROL:

4. SUPPORT:

5. RELATIONSHIPS:

6. ROLE:

7. CHANGE:

they are working effectively. Causes of stress can change and these changes need to be identified and acted upon.

Monitoring can be carried out by using two distinct methods, qualitative and quantitative.

- **Qualitative methods**
  - ☐ Observation of team dynamics and working procedures
  - ☐ Discussions with individuals
  - ☐ Consultation at team meetings
- **Quantitative methods**
  - ☐ Fewer accidents/significant events
  - ☐ Lower absenteeism/sickness
  - ☐ Fewer customer/patient complaints
  - ☐ Achievement of target/goals
  - ☐ Proof of continuing professional development (certificates, etc.)

Support for individuals

It might not always be possible to prevent an individual from suffering a stress-related illness. Once it has been identified that a person is suffering from stress it is important to manage the process effectively to aid recovery. The individual could be given alternative duties for a period of time or they may need to be on sick leave. The following process should take place in order to ensure that the individual's return to his/her normal duties or back-to-work process runs smoothly and helps rebuild his/her confidence.

- The employer should maintain contact with the employee to offer supports and to show they care.
- Determine the need for a health assessment and offer help from outside agencies and assist with the referral process.
- Agree on a suitable return-to-duties or return-to-work programme which includes a measured transition.
- Monitor and review the transition to ensure that it meets the needs and revise if necessary.

Summary

Stress can cause serious health problems and if not recognised could have a detrimental effect on individuals and the organisation. Through an effective stress management policy, suitable and sufficient risk assessment and applying the HSE's management standards, an organisation can prevent or greatly reduce the risk of stress.

Action – check the following

- Do you have a stress management policy that acknowledges the importance of identifying and reducing workplace stressors?
- Do you have systems in place for individuals to raise concerns?
- Have you carried out a work-related stress risk assessment?
- Are you applying the HSE's Management Standards to reduce the risk of stress in your organisation?

Frequently asked questions

Q. What occupations are more susceptible to stress?

A. It is possible that occupations where employees are dealing with the public are more likely to be stressful than some other occupations. Examples of such occupations are as follows:

- ☐ Teachers.
- ☐ Carers and social workers who deal with attitudes and behaviours.
- ☐ Those who deal with major accidents will be affected by the devastation of what they experience.
- ☐ Anyone who has to meet strict deadlines and targets may also be more susceptible.

Q. Can an employer insist that a sufferer seeks the help of a counsellor?

A. The employer should have a stress policy that demonstrates his/her commitment to dealing with work-related stress. Risk assessments will show that this commitment is being implemented through risk control. The referral to specialist help can be seen as a last resort where all other measures have been unsuccessful. The employer cannot insist that a sufferer seeks the help of a counsellor, but can explain the benefits that this intervention could bring.

Links to other chapters

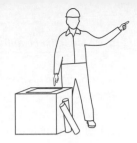

21 Visitors, locums and contractors

Scope of this chapter

- Principles of safe working practices
- Legislation
- Roles and responsibilities
- Visitors
- Locums (temporary staff)
- Contractors

Figures

Principles of safe working practices

As discussed throughout this manual, the health and safety of anyone entering the premises must be managed 'so far as is reasonably practicable'. You will already have systems and procedures in place to safeguard and therefore protect your permanent employees and your patients. However, there are additional factors to consider for visitors, locums (temporary staff) and contractors.

Legislation

- Health and Safety at Work etc. Act 1974:

  Employers and controllers of premises are required to ensure, so far as is reasonably practicable, the health, safety and welfare of all employees and protecting persons other than those at work against risks to health and safety arising out of or in connection with the activities of persons at work.

- Management of Health and Safety at Work Regulations 1999:

  Employers to make suitable and sufficient assessments of risks to health and safety of employees and persons not in his employment to identify the measures needed to remove the risks or reduce to an acceptable level and set up effective management systems to prevent and protect all those who may be affected.

- The Occupiers' Liability Act 1957 and 1984:

  The Act places a duty on occupiers, in terms of civil liability, to take reasonable care of visitors who are invited to or permitted on their premises. Visiting children should be expected to be less careful than adults. This duty extends to unlawful visitors, for example trespassers if the occupier is aware of the danger.

- Conduct of Employment Agencies and Employment Businesses Regulations 2003:

  The 'hirer', person/host organisation who the temporary worker is supplied to, should take into consideration that the locum will be unfamiliar with the premises and safety procedures within the organisation.

- Construction (Design and Management) Regulations 2007 (CDM 2007):

  The employer referred to as the Client, should ensure that construction work does not start until the competency of those involved has been assessed and a health and safety plan is in place.

Roles and responsibilities

Individuals have a common duty of care to protect those who may be affected by their activities. It is essential people understand their shared duties and are made aware of their responsibilities at the start of the visit or prior to commencement of any work. Cooperation between all parties is an essential aspect of health and safety management and should be a two-way process. In this chapter, we will address the health and safety management and shared responsibilities of all parties concerned.

Visitors

This section does not relate to patients as you will already have a system in place to keep track of who is attending for dental treatment and when they arrive and leave. If your practice is safe for employees then it should be safe for visitors. However, there are separate arrangements that should be in place for visitors as they will be unfamiliar with the workplace and emergency procedures. The following procedure should be carried out from the start of the visit until they leave your premises.

- Establish identity of person, who they are representing and ask for identification.

- Confirm purpose of visit and person they are visiting.
- Ask them to complete a visitors' book or issue a visitors' pass (Figure 21.1).
  - □ Please note that a visitors' book does not ensure confidentiality of information; therefore, a visitors' pass may be more appropriate.
- Provide a safety card (Figure 21.2).
- Briefly inform them of safety arrangements (reinforce contents of Figures 21.1 and 21.2).
- Tell them about restricted areas and what amenities are available, for example, toilets.
- Inform them of any 'special arrangements' applicable to the purpose of their visit.
- Assign someone to be responsible for the visitor.
- Supervise/accompany visitors at all times for their safety.
- Inform and train staff routinely on how to manage the evacuation of visitors (consider people with special needs, e.g. disabled visitors) and how to deal with those who enter restricted or prohibited areas.
- If construction work is taking place at the time of the visit, provide the visitor with the necessary personal protective equipment (PPE) as identified in the risk assessment.
- Ensure visitors 'sign out' or return the visitors' pass to reception before leaving.
- All of the above should be an arrangement in Part 3 of your Health and Safety Policy.

Visitors should be provided with information on any health and safety risks and the control measures designed to protect them, and should be informed about emergency procedures. Signs and notices should be displayed in prominent places so that they are clearly visible to visitors.

Locums (temporary staff)

Locums are those who are not part of your permanent workforce but who work on your premises and carry out the agreed work activities. They could be contracted from an employment agency, employment business or independently. Regardless of where they are contracted from, information should be collected and shared to ensure their health and safety and that of anyone who

VISITORS' PASS	Visitor/Pass number:
Visitor's Name:	
Company:	
Visiting:	
Time in:	Time out:
Vehicle registration:	Date:
Please return this pass to reception after use, thank you	

Side 2

Visitors – Please read carefully
1. Practice Health and Safety Policy applies to all visitors
2. FIRE/EMERGENCY – On hearing the fire alarm, leave the building by the nearest exit
3. CAR PARKING – Vehicles and contents are left at owners risk
4. SUPERVISION – You will be accompanied at all times while in the building
5. RESTRICTED ACCESS – Visitors must not enter certain areas
6. PERSONAL PROTECTION – Visitors may be required to wear PPE
7. Please sign out and return the pass to reception before leaving the building

Figure 21.1   Visitors' pass.

might be affected by their activities. The following process should be carried out:

Selecting locums

- Criminal Records Bureau (CRB) and Independent Safeguarding Authority (ISA) disclosure check should be undertaken (not yet mandatory for all dental professionals).
  - Created to help prevent unsuitable people working with children and vulnerable adults
- Confirmation of any relevant qualifications, claims to competence and insurances/professional indemnity.
- Evidence of continuing professional development (CPD) in line with General Dental Council (GDC) requirements.

- Information regarding any medical conditions that could put them or others at risk (information supplied must be used only for the purpose of the appointment).
- Verification of immunisation status.
- Information on relevant risks and controls in place, any specific tasks you may want them to do and additional skills required of the locum.

Working with locums

- A person should be assigned to supervise/mentor/buddy the locum.
- Induction should cover the main elements of health and safety essentials as follows:
  - Accident reporting procedure and first aid provision

□ Fire safety – action on discovering a fire, hearing the fire alarm, evacuation procedure routes and exits
□ Other emergency arrangements, that is, power failure and bomb threat
□ PPE/C required
□ How to use work equipment safely including computers
□ Safe movement of loads and people
□ Radiation protection (Quality Assurance Manual)
□ Safety of hazardous substances
■ Understanding and agreement of the above should be confirmed.
■ The hirer/host employer is responsible for reporting accidents involving locums under The Reporting of Injuries, Diseases and Dangerous Occurrences Regulations 1995 (RIDDOR).

Communication between all parties is essential to ensure their safety. If the locum is with you for some time you may need to refresh the above-mentioned procedures.

Contractors

There is a link between the previous section on locums and this section. Contractors are people who are not employed at the practice but brought in to carry out work on the premises. Contractors could be cleaning staff (from an agency) or window cleaners who carry out work on a regular basis; maintenance engineers from a supply company; a supplier of training/consultancy service or a construction company. The health and safety arrangements or safety contract will vary depending on the actual work they are undertaking. However, the following can be applied to all situations where contractors are used. Contractors involved in carrying out construction work have specific duties to ensure the work is carried out safely; therefore, a separate section is dedicated to these workers.

Planning to work with contractors

As the 'client' you are required to ensure the project/job is managed effectively and safely.

■ Identify all aspects of the job you want undertaken and decide how it will affect the day-to-day operations of the practice.
■ Determine what the risks are while the work is being carried out and who will be affected.
■ Identify who will manage the project/job and liaise/communicate with the contractor/s and your employees.

Selecting a contractor

The cooperation of contractors is vital to the health and safety of your practice and you need to ensure that they will comply with your safety arrangements and standards.

■ Search the Health and Safety Executive (HSE) Enforcement database for any prosecutions and notices – www.hse.gov.uk (alphabetical search, E = Enforcement).
■ Obtain copies of their Public Liability/Employers Liability Insurance certificate, Health and Safety Policy/Procedures, method statement (see definition) and generic risk assessments.
   □ Method statement – describes how the contractor is going to carry out the job with safety in mind, including what PPE will be worn, what safe systems of work will be implemented, how they will control all operations, what equipment will be used, how work will be timetabled and any emergency procedures that may be appropriate.
■ Gather information on accidents/incidents they have had and how these were acted upon.
■ Establish if they are going to use subcontractors. If so, what is their selection criteria and how can they prove that any migrant workers are working here legally, that is, using identity cards.
■ Ask if they are members of any trade organisations.

Before work starts

It is important that you (the client) allow time to plan the project in hand as this will facilitate the coordination of the entire project and allow for

VISITOR SAFETY (Green)

Visitors must keep to the designated areas (Blue)

Health and Safety at
Work Act 1974
Persons entering these premises
must comply with all safety
regulations under the above act

Visitors must not enter the restricted areas (Red)

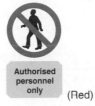

Authorised
personnel
only   (Red)

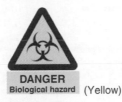

DANGER
Biological hazard   (Yellow)

CAUTION
Radiation
area   (Yellow)

Visitors must wear appropriate PPE in certain areas (Blue)

Eye protection
must be worn

Side 2

FIRE ROUTINE (Blue)

IF YOU DISCOVER A FIRE
- Operate the nearest Fire Alarm Call Point
- Do not tackle the fire or take personal risks
- Evacuate the building by the safest route
- Report to assembly point which is:.........................
IF YOU HEAR THE FIRE ALARM
- Leave the building by the safest route
- Close all doors behind you
- Report to assembly point which is:.........................

DO NOT (Red)
- Use lifts
- Stop to collect personal belongings
- Re-enter the building until authorised to do so

Figure 21.2 Safety card.

all foreseeable occurrences. The following should be undertaken:

- The contractor must carry out a risk assessment covering all aspects of the job.
- The risk assessment must then be discussed with all parties, owner/occupier and subcontractor and the control measures agreed.
- Existing practice risk assessments must also be discussed and revised if they will no longer be valid.
- Determine how the work will affect the health and safety of patients and what information they will need.

Safety management throughout the project

- All parties must communicate, consult and cooperate with each other.
- Employees should be kept informed about all aspects of the job and be provided with any necessary additional training.
- Any changes to the original job, which could render the risk assessment invalid or require it to be revised, must be identified and acted upon.
- The performance of contractors and subcontractors needs to be monitored and any concerns raised and rectified.
- All accidents and incidents must be investigated and analysed for causative factors and recurrence prevented (significant event analysis).
- If there are serious concerns, work should be stopped immediately and not restarted until a suitable solution has been determined.

Construction work

In addition to the above sections (planning and selecting contractors) the following should be carried out where any type of construction work is taking place:

- In the case of notifiable projects (see definition) appoint a competent Construction Design Management (CDM) coordinator who will advise on the appointment of suitable

contractors and assist with and coordinate health and safety arrangements.
  - □ Definition
    Notifiable project – project that lasts longer than 30 days or involves more than 500 person days of construction work. Any day on which construction work is carried out (including holidays and weekends) should be counted, even if the work on that day is of short duration. A person day is one individual, including supervisors and specialists, carrying out construction work for one normal working shift (*Source: HSE Notification of Construction Project*).
- If the work is classed as a Notifiable Project, a form F10 must be sent to the enforcing authority as soon as possible after the CDM coordinator has been selected. Form F10 provides comprehensive details covering all aspects of the project and any additions must be subsequently notified.
- Appoint a Principal Contractor (the CDM coordinator will advise on a suitable person or act as same) to plan and manage the work and prepare the health and safety plan before work starts. The health and safety file should be prepared, renewed or updated ready for handover at the end of the project.
- Ask the contractor for evidence of belonging to Construction Skills Certification Scheme (CSCS) as this confirms occupational competence.

Summary

Employers are responsible for the health and safety of all persons who may be affected by their activities; this includes all those mentioned in this chapter. Measures must be taken to avoid people being exposed to risks which could have a detrimental effect on their health and safety.

Action – check the following

- Do you have an arrangement in Part 3 of your Health and Safety Policy to manage the health and safety of visitors, locums and contractors?

- Do you provide sufficient information for visitors to ensure their safety while on the premises?
- Are your induction procedures suitable and sufficient for locums?
- Have you selected competent contractors and are you confident they will carry out work safely?
- Do you have a list of 'preferred contractors' who have demonstrated safe working practices and whom you use frequently?

Frequently asked questions

Q. What is meant by the term 'reasonably practicable'?

A. This is a legal term which allows a cost-benefit analysis to be used when determining what is reasonable within the circumstances in response to an identified risk.

Q. If patients are not required to complete the visitors' book or pass, how should we best manage their safety while they are on the premises?

A. Patients will be supervised and chaperoned for the majority of time; therefore, they will not be left unattended. Ensure evacuation notices are prominently displayed in waiting and reception areas and train staff on evacuating patients quickly and safely without causing unnecessary panic or alarming them.

Q. Do we have to provide personal protective equipment for locum staff?

A. Under the Health and Safety at Work etc. Act 1974 it is the duty of employers to conduct undertakings in such a way as to ensure, so far as is reasonable, that persons not in their employment who may be affected are not exposed to risks to their health and safety. Therefore, the hirer/host employer may need to provide PPE to comply with this duty.

Q. If someone trips over something that a contractor has left on the floor, who is liable?

A. It is your duty to select contractors who will not put people at risk. Someone could make a claim against your liability insurance. It would then be your responsibility to demonstrate that you were not negligent. This gives emphasis to the importance of appointing competent contractors and monitoring their work.

Q. What constitutes construction work?

A. Construction work includes a range of activities, for example, alterations, conversions, renovations, repairs, maintenance, redecoration and demolition, to mention just a few.

Links to other chapters

- Chapter 3 – Communication and training
- Chapter 11 – Lone working
- Chapter 17 – Policy
- Chapter 19 – Risk assessment
- Chapter 23 – Working environment

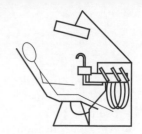

22 Work equipment

Scope of this chapter

- Introduction
- Legislation
- Range of work equipment
- Hazards associated with work equipment
- General safety requirements
- Dentistry-specific safety requirements

Figures

Introduction

Work equipment is found in every dental practice and includes any machinery, appliance, apparatus, tool, installation, instrument and any assembly that is used by people to carry out their work. Work equipment can present risks to users, if not used correctly or maintained in safe working order. The nature and significance of the risk associated with this equipment depends on the following factors:

- The type of activity/task undertaken
- The type of equipment used
- The purpose of the equipment
- The number of people involved in the activity/task
- The competence of staff

This chapter provides general and specific legislative and good practice requirements in order to facilitate compliance. The general principles of safety can be applied to all equipment used in dental practices, although some equipment requires specific arrangements to be in place. Regardless of the type of equipment used general safety measures must be applied in all cases. The measures apply to new and second-hand equipment purchased and equipment hired or leased for use at work.

Legislation

- Health and Safety at Work etc. Act 1974:

  Employers have a duty to ensure, so far as is reasonably practicable, the provision and maintenance of plant and equipment that is safe and without risks to health.

- Provision and Use of Work Equipment Regulations 1998 (PUWER):

Employers are required to provide and maintain safe equipment and safe working procedures to ensure that work is carried out safely.

- Management of Health and Safety at Work Regulations 1999:

Employers must assess the risks to employees' health and safety from the use of work equipment. Eliminate the risks where reasonable or reduce to an acceptable level. Employees must use work equipment as trained and instructed to ensure its safe use.

- Electricity at Work Regulations 1989:

Employers must ensure that all electrical systems, including high voltage to battery-operated equipment, is constructed and maintained to prevent the risk of injury arising out of work activities.

- Pressure Safety Systems Regulations 2000:

Employers are required to ensure that pressure vessels are used in line with safe operating limits and pressure and temperature requirements and there is a written scheme of examination in place.

- Medical Devices Regulations 2002 (as amended):

Employers are required to have a system in place to manage the purchase, use and maintenance of medical devices to ensure that all risks, so far as is reasonable, are reduced.

- Lifting Operations and Lifting Equipment Regulations 1998 (LOLER):

Employers must ensure that lifting equipment is of adequate strength and stability for the load that is to be lifted, in particular equipment used for lifting persons must consider the operator and the person being carried.

- Carriage of Dangerous Goods and Use of Transportable Pressure Equipment Regulations 2009:

Employers have a duty to provide a safe place of work where a pressure receptacle is being used, to ensure the equipment is in safe working order and to design and implement a safe system of work.

- Personal Protective Equipment at Work Regulations 1992 (as amended 2002):

Employers are required to select, provide and maintain suitable PPE and to ensure appropriate use, where risks cannot be adequately controlled by any other means.

Range of work equipment

In dentistry, the range of equipment is vast; however, it can be consolidated into two groups, namely equipment and instruments. Equipment is fixed or portable and manually or power operated. Examples of both groups appear below:

- Decontamination equipment
- Dental chair, unit and light
- Disposables
- Gas cylinders
- Hand-held dental instruments
- Office equipment
- Portable electrical appliances
- Pressure vessels
- Radiography equipment
- Rotary or air-driven instruments
- Suction units

The above is not an exhaustive list as it is impractical to list everything. However, the requirements of the Provision and Use of Work Equipment Regulations and other associated legislation must be applied to everything that comes under the definition of work equipment.

Hazards associated with work equipment

An appreciation of the hazards presented by work equipment is important in order to effectively implement the safety precautions. The hazards range from relatively minor consequences to more serious and, in some cases, potentially fatal ones. The following list provides an overview of the more generic hazards:

- Electric shock
- Fire
- Faulty design or installation
- Entanglement with moving parts
- Entrapment from equipment falling over
- Impact from the release of particles ejecting
- Biological, chemical or radioactive contamination
- Noise or vibration
- Dusts, vapours or fumes
- Burns or scalds from contact with heating systems
- Transmission of infectious disease through sharps
- Upper limb disorder from poor posture
- Uncontrollable release of stored energy under pressure resulting in explosion

Everyone is exposed to the above hazards; therefore, the safety of users, operators, others in the immediate vicinity and the outcome of instrument malfunction or failure which may adversely affect patient care must be addressed.

General safety requirements

As you will see from the 'legislation' section in this chapter there is a wide range of regulations which apply to work equipment and some will overlap. In order to prevent repetition and unnecessary duplication of information, this section will address general safety requirements as contained in PUWER. Safety must be considered in three stages.

1. Purchasing (new or second hand) or leasing or hiring

- Review existing risk assessments to identify any additional risks that new equipment may present.

- Revise existing risk assessment or undertake a new one.
- Consider design, intended use and suitability of positioning/location.
- Consider any environmental contamination from the equipment and means of ventilation.
- Obtain information from manufacturers and suppliers on design safety features.
- Check whether equipment is manufactured to the European standard and displays the CE mark and whether an EC declaration of conformity certificate is issued (if required) or
- If manufactured prior to 1995, it is safe for use.
- Safe operating information and instruction manual is provided.
- Confirm that manufacturer or supplier maintenance and testing schedules will be undertaken as and when required.
- Consider competencies of those using equipment and identify training needs.
- Ensure that equipment is safe and suitable for its purpose.

2. Using

- Prior to an employee using new or existing equipment, a risk assessment should be undertaken as follows:
  □ Identify hazards – look at the activity which involves the use of the equipment and identify any hazards that may be present (use the previous section for a range of hazards).
  □ Evaluate the risks – determine who is exposed to the equipment and therefore could be harmed, how the harm may arise, for example, steam emits from autoclave when door is opened. Identify how the risks are currently being controlled and are they sufficient and then determine the overall severity of the risk.
  □ Implement additional controls – if additional controls are required the hierarchy approach should be adopted (see Chapter 19). Control measures should address the equipment, working practices and competence of users. An example is

provided in relation to X-ray processing equipment.

◻ Manual 3-tank X-ray processing equipment
  • Substitute the equipment for an automatic processor.
  • Ensure equipment is used in well-ventilated area, is turned off when not in use and inspected and tested annually.
  • Provide training on safe use and routine maintenance of equipment.

◻ Monitor control measures – periodically check that the additional control measures are effective and reduce risks; revise controls if necessary.

◻ Review risk assessments – if new equipment is purchased, if monitoring identifies that the controls are ineffective or if significant changes occur.

The risk assessment templates in Chapter 19 can be used to carry out the above. In addition to the risk assessment, the following should also be considered:

■ Safe operating procedures/method of work should be an outcome of risk assessment and made available to users.
■ All those who use, supervise or manage work equipment should be suitably informed, instructed and trained to an appropriate level.
■ Supervision should be increased for those who may be more at risk, for example, trainees/young persons.
■ Access to dangerous parts of the equipment should be guarded as appropriate.
■ Emergency stop devices should be located close to the equipment.
■ Energy isolation devices should be as appropriate, for example, cut-off valves for water and air.
■ Suitable and sufficient lighting should be provided and adequate space should be available to use equipment safely.
■ Markings and signs should be displayed where necessary, for example, ionising radiation controlled area.
■ Personal protective equipment/clothing (PPE/C) should be provided if necessary.
■ A planned inspection, testing and maintenance schedule should be in place.

3. Maintenance

Maintenance is vitally important not only for the safety of people but also to ensure that the equipment performs to the required standard and therefore is efficient. Not all equipment will need a formal system of planned maintenance; however, general requirements apply as follows:

■ Information on inspection, testing and maintenance should be obtained from the following sources:
  ◻ Manufacturers and suppliers of equipment
  ◻ Regulations, guidance and approved code of practice (ACOP)
  ◻ Professional bodies
  ◻ Industry standards
■ All equipment, powered and non-powered, should be inspected, tested and maintained in accordance with the manufacturer's, supplier's or installer's recommendations.
■ Practices should draw up an appropriate schedule of all equipment that requires maintenance (Figure 22.1 and Figure 23.2).
■ All fixed equipment should be visually inspected periodically and results recorded (Figure 23.3).
■ All portable electrical appliances should be visually inspected periodically and results recorded (Figure 22.2).
■ Information and instruction should be provided to those who undertake maintenance and their understanding and agreement confirmed.
■ Where inspection and testing is required, this should be undertaken by a competent person and outcomes recorded.
■ Maintenance programmes should be reviewed periodically and if necessary revised.
■ Maintenance procedures should be carried out without risks to a person's health or safety and in a suitable location.
■ A system should be in place to remove faulty or damaged equipment from operation until repaired or disposed of (Figure 22.3).

Air conditioning units

From January 2009, all systems over 250 kW are required to be inspected annually by an accredited air conditioning system energy assessor for

Figure 22.1 Portable appliance inspection and testing schedule.

SCHEDULE NO:			DATE	FROM:			TO:			

Equipment and location	Person/Company responsible	Frequency	Date planned	Date completed	Date planned	Date completed	Date planned	Date completed

Figure 22.2   Portable electrical appliance visual inspection.

PLEASE NOTE: The term 'Inspection' refers to a visual method only; no attempt must be made to examine the equipment by any other means. The plug should be inspected both internally and externally by removing the plug screws (if competent to do so).

DATE:			PERSON RESPONSIBLE:		
TYPE OF APPLIANCE:			LOCATION:		
FREQUENCY (CIRCLE)		WEEKLY	MONTHLY	OTHER (SPECIFY)	

No	Requirement	Yes	No	Defect/Action	Done
1. Cable					
a.	Cable covering free from cuts/abrasions				
b.	Cable joints are adequate for appliance				
c.	Cable is free of taped joints				
d.	Cable is free from contamination				
e.	Cable fits secure to appliance				
f.	Cable is correct for appliance				
2. Plug					
a.	Plug is free of burn or scorch marks				
b.	Plug is free from cracks				
c.	Plug pins are free from damage				
d.	Plug is correctly fused				
e.	Plug is free from internal damage				
f.	Wires attached to correct terminals				
g.	Terminal screws are tight				
h.	Cable grip holds outer sheath securely				
3. Appliance					
a.	Outer casing free from damage				
b.	Screws present and tight				
c.	Outer casing is free from contamination				
d.	Switches/controls functioning correctly				
e.	Protective guard functioning correctly				
f.	Valid test sticker is on appliance				
g.	Appliance has the CE mark				
h.	Appliance suitable for the environment				
4. Other (if applicable)					
a.	Socket adaptors eliminated from use				
b.	Extension lead discouraged (or)				
c.	Extension lead correct for appliance				

Figure 22.3   Damaged equipment report.

Equipment is not to be used

Equipment type/name:	Equipment number: (if applicable)
Location of equipment:	Rejected by:
Date rejected:	Reported to:

Reasons for rejection:

Action taken (1a or 2a or 3a)		
1a. Sent for repair (specify repairer)	2a. Disposed/removed (by whom)	3a. Other (please specify)
1b. Repairs carried out (date)	2b. Equipment removed (date)	3b. Other carried out (date)

Any other comments:

energy efficiency. The requirement is part of the European Union's Energy Performance in Building Directive (EPBD). By January 2011, all air conditioning systems over 12 kW must have had their first annual inspection. Also from 2011, if a person in control of the air conditioning system changes, and an inspection report is not forwarded to the successor, the person now responsible for air conditioning must commission an inspection within 3 months (*Source: Delphos Project Services Ltd*).

The general safety requirements listed above will also apply to medical devices as contained in the next section.

Dentistry-specific safety requirements

A large amount of equipment and instruments used in dental practices are classed as 'Medical Devices'. The term *medical device* is defined as:

Any device, instrument, apparatus, appliance, software, material or other article, whether used alone or in combination, together with any accessory, including the software intended by its manufacturer to be used for human beings specifically for diagnosis or therapeutic purposes or both and necessary for its proper application.

The use, care and maintenance of all medical devices must adhere to the instructions given by the manufacturer or supplier. In addition, infection control must be considered in all instances. This section addresses the use and maintenance of some of the medical devices.

Gas cylinders

- Take care when handling to prevent the cylinder being dropped and the risk of manual handling injuries.
- Do not lift the cylinder by the cap which protects the valve and do not drag or roll them.
- Store cylinders upright and ensure that they are stable and cannot fall over.
- Store and use in a well-ventilated area away from direct sunlight and clearly marked with appropriate signs.

- Do not allow grease or oil to come in contact with the valves; it may result in explosion.
- Do not place near naked flame as heat can damage it.
- Ensure cylinders are labelled, and familiarise yourself with the content.
- When opening valves stand to the side, not directly in front of the valve.
- When cylinders are not in use valves must be closed.
- Ensure you are competent to assist with the use of gas cylinders for all procedures.
- Removal of gas cylinders from the practice must be by an authorised company.
- In addition to the above, safety considerations are covered in Chapter 9.

Never use compressed gases or compressed air to clean dust or other substances from clothing; air may enter the eyes or the body tissues.

Hand instruments

- Ensure that all instruments are decontaminated in line with Health Technical Memorandum (HTM) 01-05.
- Handle instruments safely to prevent the risk of inoculation injury.
- Allow instruments to cool after sterilisation before touching.
- Visually check instruments routinely for wear and tear and replace components when necessary.
- Use appropriate devices to sharpen instruments.
- Ensure that hinges and joints on instruments move freely and lubricate according to manufacturer's instructions.
- Store instruments securely to prevent damage.
- Dispose of damaged instruments in line with Hazardous Waste Regulations.
- Equipment labelled as single use must only be used for a single procedure and disposed of in line with Hazardous Waste Regulations.

Handpieces and air-driven instruments

- Carry out routine maintenance, decontamination and lubrication in line with manufacturer's instructions.

- Do not place handpieces in an ultrasonic bath or under water.
- Water lines for handpieces should be run through immediately before use to prevent back-syphoning.
- Ensure scaling tips are covered or placed downwards when on the dental unit to prevent inoculation injury.
- Sterilise instruments with lumens in a vacuum autoclave if possible.

Pressure vessels

Autoclaves

- A written scheme of examination must be in place before the autoclave is in operation; initial testing and inspection must be undertaken by a competent engineer.
- The pressure vessel must be examined in accordance with the written scheme of examination.
- Periodic examination should be carried out by a competent engineer at least once in every 14 months for steam-generating autoclaves and every 26 months for other types (unless specified otherwise). Examination should pay particular attention to functioning of all safety devices, safety interlocks and fittings.
- Appropriate PPE must be worn when using and carrying out routine maintenance.
- Carry out routine daily maintenance (Figure 22.4) as follows:
  - □ Wipe door seals, fill up water reservoir (check with manufacturer's guidelines for water type), place process indicator strip on tray, close door and start a normal cycle (check with manufacturer's guidelines if this should be with or without a load).
  - □ [1]Record the following details (if autoclave has a recorder or printer examine the record for compliance):
    - Date, time, serial number and location of unit
    - Cycle counter number
    - Time to reach holding temperature

- Temperature during holding period[1]
- Pressure during holding period[1]
- Total time at holding temperature/pressure
- Water drained at end of previous day
- Name/s of authorised user/s
- Door seals secure
- Door safety devices functioning correctly
- Any comments
- Name and signature of tester
  - □ If the following conditions are achieved the autoclave can be used:
    - 'Cycle complete' signal is visible.
    - Record shows cycle temperatures and pressures are within expectations.
    - Door could not be operated until 'cycle complete' signal is visible.
    - There are no abnormalities.

Autoclaves must be used and maintained in line with the appropriate regulations and the HTM 01-05 and appropriate records held.

Compressors

Carry out routine maintenance in line with manufacturer's instructions. This will differ depending on the make and model; the following instructions relate to a particular model:

- Do not touch the compressor during operation.
- Keep flammable substances away from direct contact.
- Carry out weekly maintenance as follows:
  - □ Check oil gauge levels.
  - □ Empty the drain bottle.
  - □ Drain water tank.
  - □ Drain filter valve.
  - □ Ensure the fan at the top of the cover is working, fan starts when the motor reaches a specific temperature and runs until the temperature drops.
- Carry out monthly maintenance as follows:
  - □ Check compressor air tubes and equipment for leaks and check the pumping time.
  - □ Inspect and replace filter if necessary.
  - □ Clean compressor with a damp, soft cloth to remove dust and debris which may prevent cooling.

---

[1] Only applicable if autoclave has temperature/pressure displays/gauges.

Figure 22.4 Daily autoclave test.

DATE: TIME:

SERIAL NUMBER: LOCATION:

Activity	Observe	Evidence		Comment or action
1.	Cycle counter number			
2.	Time to reach holding temperature			
3.	Temperature during holding period*			
4.	Pressure during holding period*			
5.	Total time at holding temperature			
6.	Water drained at end of previous day	Yes	No	
7.	Name/s of authorised user/s			
8.	Door seals secure	Yes	No	
9.	Door safety devices functioning correctly	Yes	No	
10.	Any comments:			
11.	Name of tester:	Signature of tester:		
Additional comments:				

*Applicable only if autoclave has temperature/pressure displays/gauges. Please attach each TST (time, steam and temperature) strip to this test sheet.

In addition to the above, annual maintenance must be carried out by a competent engineer and usually involves the following:

☐ Check the O-ring in the non-return valve and replace if necessary.
☐ Empty receiver of air before dismounting.
☐ Check filter and elements.
☐ Test the safety valve by gently pulling the ring with pressure in the receiver.

Suction systems

■ Waste into the main drainage system must comply with local water/sewage regulations.
■ Use correct solution as recommended; solutions must be CE marked.
■ Systems must be 'aspirated through' daily at the end of a session; in some instances, for example, for prolonged surgical procedures, twice daily may be required.

- Maintenance should involve a two-stage approach:
  □ Stage 1 – aspirate through with a biodegradable non-foaming agent.
  □ Stage 2 – aspirate through with an appropriate disinfectant.
- Where amalgam separators are not fitted filters should be removed, contents disposed of appropriately and cleaned before repositioning.
- Heavy duty gloves, masks, eye protection and plastic aprons should be worn.

Amalgam separators

- Determine if waste amalgam collection allows that which is from the separator.
- Frequency and nature of maintenance will depend on the type of separator installed; for example, a single unit separator may require more frequent maintenance owing to its 'serving' a number of surgeries.

Ultrasonic bath

- Fill bath to recommended level with appropriate solution and water.
- Place rinsed instruments in basket, submerge in bath and replace the lid.
- Switch on bath and set timer as recommended.
- When cycle is complete remove basket and rinse instruments.
- Visually check for debris; if no debris, dry and place in autoclave; if debris is visible repeat the process.
- Do not turn bath on when empty of water.
- Drain bath at end of day or when contaminated.
- Carry out 'soil test' regularly to monitor optimum cleaning times.
- Wear appropriate PPE when using and maintaining bath.

Washer disinfectors

- Carry out routine maintenance in line with manufacturer's instructions.

- Ensure that instruments can be decontaminated in wet heat at high temperatures.
- Ensure that installation is suitable in the setting; for example, water supply and electrical power is reliable.
- Temperature measurements must be achieved and held at the pre-set temperature for the required holding time in order to reach all areas of the chamber.
- Chamber cycle parameters should be checked routinely.
- Loads must be visually checked after a cycle to ensure effective cleaning.
- Cleaning efficiency and thermometric checks should be carried out in line with manufacturer's instruction.
- Appropriate PPE must be worn.

Lifting equipment

In some dental settings, hoists are used to move physically disabled patients into the dental chair. The regulations place specific duties on employers to ensure that equipment is used safely without risks to the operator and the person being lifted. The lifting equipment must

- be installed and positioned in a safe area;
- be stable and capable of carrying the weight it is intended for;
- prevent the user from being trapped, crushed or struck by the equipment;
- not expose the person being carried to any danger;
- have a plan in place in the event of an emergency;
- have a scheduled system of maintenance.

Summary

Employers must select work equipment with safety in mind, consider suitable location and installation and always have safe working procedures to hand to ensure its safe operation. Identify training needs of staff and carry out planned service and maintenance procedures in line with manufacturer's instructions. Ensure that work equipment meets the EU standards and displays the CE mark where appropriate.

Action – check the following

- Do you have a planned maintenance schedule in place for equipment?
- Do you routinely carry out visual inspections on all equipment?
- Do you identify training needs of all staff to ensure that equipment is used safely?

Frequently asked questions

Q. When inspecting and testing electrical equipment does the person have to be a qualified electrician?

A. The person undertaking the maintenance must be competent, he/she must have working knowledge of electricity and be able to understand hazards associated with the equipment. In addition, if the equipment is faulty the person should be able to interpret the fault and rectify it, so that it is safe to take it out or use.

Q. Do portable appliances have to be tested every year?

A. Not necessarily; you need to consider what the appliance is used for and where, the frequency of use, how often it is moved to other areas, the likelihood of it becoming damaged and where it is stored. This will help you to determine the frequency of testing; the HSE provides a guide to the frequency of inspection and testing; this can be found in Chapter 7.

Links to other chapters

Chapter 6 – Display screen equipment
Chapter 7 – Electrical safety
Chapter 9 – Hazardous substances
Chapter 10 – Infection control
Chapter 16 – Personal protective equipment
Chapter 18 – Radiation protection
Chapter 19 – Risk assessment

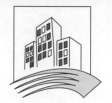

23 Working environment

Scope of this chapter

- Introduction
- Legislation
- Responsibilities
- Safe workplace principles
- Working from home

Figures

Introduction

Workplace is defined as any premises or part of premises which are made available to any person as a place of work. It also includes any part of the premises that employees have access to while at work, for example, corridor, staircase, entrance and exit. If an employee is working from home this also comes under the definition and the risks associated must be addressed.

Legislation

- Workplace (Health, Safety and Welfare) Regulations 1992:

  Every employer shall ensure that the health and safety of everyone is protected and that adequate welfare facilities are provided for people at work. Every workplace that is under his control and where any of his employees' work, is maintained in an efficient state and in good repair.

- Health and Safety at Work etc. Act 1974:

  Employers must maintain a safe place of work, with safe access and egress, a safe working environment with adequate welfare facilities.

- The Health and Safety (Signs and Signals) Regulations 1996:

  Employers are required to use safety signs and appropriate signals where significant risks exist which cannot be controlled by any other means.

Managing Health and Safety in the Dental Practice: A Practical Guide, by Jane Bonehill   © 2010 by Blackwell Publishing Ltd.

- Work at Height Regulations 2005 (as amended 2007):

  Employers are required to assess the risks associated with working at heights and eliminate the task where possible. If it is not possible then control measures should be implemented to prevent people from falling.

- Construction (Design and Management) Regulations 2007 (CDM 2007):

  The Client, this could be owner/occupier, must ensure, before work starts, that all construction work is adequately controlled. Designers of workplaces are required to ensure that risks are designed out of the workplace/ building.

- Disability Discrimination Act 1995 (as amended 2005):

  Employers/Occupiers/Owners must make reasonable adjustments to the physical features of premises to overcome barriers to access to the services.

- Occupiers' Liability Act 1957 and 1984:

  Occupiers of premises must take reasonable care for the safety of visitors to their premises. The duty of care extends to trespassers if the occupier for example is aware of the danger.

Responsibilities

Employers

- They are required to ensure that the workplace is safe and healthy for employees and anyone else who may be affected including visitors/patients, including safe access to, and egress from, the premises.
- They are required to ensure that the activities undertaken are, so far as is reasonable, controlled to reduce the risk of injury to any persons.
- They are required to provide employees and visitors/patients with information and instruction – for example, the use of safety signs and signals. The colour and shape of the sign identifies its category. The main categories of safety signs are as follows:
  - Warning – triangular, black pictogram on yellow background – for hazards, that is, flammable materials, ionising radiation controlled area
  - Mandatory – round, white pictogram on blue background – telling people they must do something, that is, wear protective clothing
  - Prohibition – round, red pictogram on white background – prohibiting certain activities, that is, smoking
  - Safe condition – rectangular, white pictogram on green background – giving information about safety features such as fire exit routes
- They are required to undertake suitable and sufficient risk assessments to identify hazards, evaluate risks and implement control measures.
- They should restrict public access to hazardous areas.
- They should ensure the internal and external maintenance of premises.
- They must ensure the safe provision and maintenance of any 'fixed equipment', for example, air conditioning and gas boilers.
- They may have other specific duties as discussed throughout this chapter.

Occupiers and those in control of premises

The following are the responsibilities in addition to the above duties:

- If the property is leased and you are the tenant ensure that the terms of the lease are agreed on before occupying the premises; it is important that you obtain this in writing. In most tenancy agreements, it is customary for the tenant to have the duty for health and safety.
- In most cases, tenants have a responsibility for internal and external maintenance and repairs.
- In shared premises, employers should cooperate with other tenants on health and safety issues and coordinate some activities, for example, fire evacuation procedures.

Employees

- Must cooperate with the employer to enable him to comply with legal duties
- Should report hazardous conditions or defects to the employer
- Should not intentionally interfere with or misuse anything that is provided for their health, safety and welfare

Public (visitors/patients)

- Should adhere to information and instruction provided by the owner/occupier. For example, they should follow instructions given on health and safety signs and signals such as fire evacuation.
- If providing assistance to a patient or a child, ensure that they take responsibility for that person or child at all times.
- Should not intentionally interfere with or damage anything that is provided.

Landlords

Responsibilities of the landlords will be dependent on the terms of the lease. However, the following provides a general guide:

- Keep the premises in a safe and habitable condition.
- Conduct electrical safety checks including wiring systems before leasing premises.
- In 'shared premises', the landlords are responsible for common parts. These are areas that are shared with other people, for example, this may include access to the premises and stairways.
- They are responsible for maintaining and checking that shared emergency equipment, for example, fire alarms and fire extinguishers on shared areas such as stairways are fit for use.
- They are responsible for lawfully evicting a tenant, by obtaining a signed court order, if the terms of the lease have been breached. An example might be if the tenant damages the premises.

- In some situations, the landlord may enlist the services of a managing agent who will act on behalf of the landlord under the terms of the lease, and will therefore have shared responsibilities.

Safe workplace principles

The following provisions are considered necessary for all dental environments which are classed as enclosed (internal) workplaces. This is not an exhaustive list and further requirements can be found in The Workplace (Health, Safety and Welfare) Regulations 1992 (as amended):

- **Maintenance of workplace, fixed equipment and systems**
  - ☐ Employers should have a planned workplace inspection schedule (Figure 23.1).
  - ☐ Employers should discuss and agree on the frequency of fixed equipment maintenance work with the appropriate maintenance company (Figure 23.2).
  - ☐ Maintenance work should routinely be carried out on all fixed equipment mentioned in this chapter and on the following:
    - Gas supply and appliances
    - Electric plug sockets
    - Emergency lighting
    - Water and air supply
    - Any other fixed equipment as deemed necessary, that is, central aspiration unit, X-ray set and central heating boiler
  - ☐ Employers should carry out routine workplace and fixed equipment inspections to confirm safe conditions or identify defects. (Figure 23.3). Please note that the inspection must be carried out by visual observation only and no attempt must be made to rectify any defects.
  - ☐ Repair and maintenance work should be carried out regularly at suitable intervals and defects rectified. While maintenance work is being carried out, access should be prevented where necessary. Records should be obtained from the person/company carrying out the work and held of all maintenance work.

Figure 23.1 Workplace inspection schedule.

SCHEDULE NO:		DATE	FROM:				TO:		
Work area	Person responsible	Frequency	Date planned	Date completed	Date planned	Date completed	Date planned	Date completed	

To be used in conjunction with Workplace and Fixed Equipment Inspection Record (Figure 23.3), for visual inspection purpose only

Figure 23.2 Fixed equipment visual inspection and maintenance schedule.

SCHEDULE NO:		DATE	FROM:			TO:			

Equipment and location	Person/Company responsible	Frequency	Date planned	Date completed	Date planned	Date completed	Date planned	Date completed

To be used in conjunction with Workplace and Fixed Equipment Inspection Record (Figure 23.3), for visual inspection purpose only

Figure 23.3   Workplace and fixed equipment inspection record.

PLEASE NOTE: The term 'Inspection' refers to a visual method only; no attempt must be made to examine an area or equipment by any other means.

DATE:	WORK AREA/S:	PERSON RESPONSIBLE:

No	Requirement	Yes	No	N/A	Defect/Action
1.	Area structurally sound				
2.	Gas appliances working effectively				
3.	Plug sockets intact and covered (where necessary)				
4.	Emergency lighting functioning correctly				
5.	Water and air supply free from leakage				
6.	All fixed equipment operating safely				
7.	Staff free from draughts and excessive air movement				
8.	Mechanical ventilation working effectively				
9.	Minimum temperatures achieved				
10.	Thermometers available				
11.	Comfortable room temperature maintained				
12.	Lighting levels sufficient and suitable				
13.	Glare from light eliminated				
14.	Light switches intact				
15.	Local lighting provided where necessary				
16.	Furniture, furnishings and fittings clean				
17.	Area clean and hygiene levels maintained				
18.	Housekeeping to the required standard				
19.	Suitable waste containers provided				
20.	Waste segregated and stored appropriately				
21.	Sufficient space to work safely				
22.	Suitable seating provided with adequate support				
23.	Work stations allow freedom of movement				
24.	Floors and corridors free from obstruction				
25.	Handrails on stairs secure				
26.	Vehicles and pedestrians segregated				
27.	Loft ladders suitable and maintained				
28.	Safe stacking and storage of objects/articles				
29.	Glass fixtures (doors/partitions) clearly marked				
30.	Doors and fittings secure and operating effectively				
31.	Windows open without risk to anyone				
32.	WC ventilated, well lit and clean				
33.	WC has soap, adequate running water and hand drying				

(continued overleaf)

Figure 23.3 *(continued)*

No	Requirement	Yes	No	N/A	Defect/Action
34.	Drinking water provided				
35.	Secure and suitable storage of clothing and personal items				
36.	Changing area fit for purpose				
37.	Rest area fit for purpose				
38.	Changing and rest areas cleaned and maintained				
39.	Disabled facilities maintained				
40.	Disabled access and egress in place and suitable				
41.	Appropriate signage displayed				

To be used in conjunction with Workplace Inspection Schedule (Figure 23.1) and Fixed Equipment Visual Inspection and Maintenance Schedule (Figure 23.2), for visual inspection purpose only

□ Employers/occupiers should ensure that people carrying out maintenance work are competent.

■ **Ventilation**
   □ There should be suitable and sufficient ventilation to allow the replacement of 'stale air'.
   □ A flow of fresh/new air (uncontaminated) should be maintained using the most suitable and effective means.
   □ Staff should not be subjected to draughts from natural or mechanical ventilation systems.
   □ Where mechanical systems are used air should be filtered, regularly cleaned, tested and maintained.

■ **Temperature**
   □ A reasonable, comfortable temperature must be maintained during working hours.
   □ Where a reasonable temperature cannot be achieved local heating or cooling should be provided.
   □ Minimum reasonable temperatures should normally be at least 16°C for dental environments.
   □ Thermometers/temperature measurement devices shall be provided to enable employees to establish the temperature.

■ **Lighting**
   □ Suitable and sufficient lighting must be provided and where possible, lighting should be natural.

□ Lighting should not produce glare on any surface, and workstations may need to be repositioned.
□ Certain areas of the building may need special consideration, for example, stairways which can cast natural shadows.
□ Local lighting should be provided where necessary at individual workstations.
□ Lighting should not be obscured, for example, by shelves or stacking systems.
□ Lights should be repaired, replaced or cleaned to maintain sufficient levels.
□ Emergency lighting should be provided where necessary and be from an independent source.

■ **Cleanliness and waste materials**
   □ Workplaces, furniture, furnishings and fittings should be kept sufficiently clean.
   □ Walls, floors and ceilings should be constructed in a material that enables effective cleaning.
   □ Effective and suitable housekeeping and cleaning should be carried out regularly to ensure that suitable hygiene levels are maintained.
   □ Spillages should be cleared up and removed as soon as possible.
   □ To reduce the risk of cross-infection, products and cleaning methods used must be appropriate to the surface and equipment being cleaned.

□ Waste materials should not accumulate to such an extent that they present a risk to a person's health. They should be appropriately segregated and stored in a suitable location.

■ **Room dimensions and space**
□ Work areas must have sufficient floor areas, height and unoccupied space for people to work safely and without risk to their health.
□ The Approved Code of Practice (ACOP) recommends 11 m^3 of workspace per person. Work equipment and furniture may need to be repositioned or relocated to achieve this space.

■ **Workstations and seating**
□ Workstations must be arranged to suit the person and the tasks being carried out.
□ Seating must be provided to suit the person using it and the tasks undertaken.
□ Seating must provide adequate support and, if necessary, a footrest if feet cannot be placed flat on the floor.
□ Workstations should allow adequate freedom of movement with sufficient clear and unobstructed space.

■ **Conditions of floor and traffic routes**
□ Floors and traffic routes (includes route for pedestrians) must be constructed bearing in mind their intended use. For example, in clinical areas, material which can be decontaminated should be used.
□ Absorbent and porous materials should be avoided in areas where there is a risk of penetration from hazardous substances.
□ Floors should be kept free from obstruction which could cause slips, trips or falls.
□ Floors should not have any unnecessary slopes, be uneven or of a slippery material.
□ Slopes or gradients should not be too steep.
□ Suitable and sufficient handrails should be placed on stairways.
□ Open sides of stairways should be securely fenced.
□ Car parks should be arranged to prevent pedestrians and vehicles from colliding.

■ **Falls and falling objects**
□ If any type of work is being carried out at a height, reasonable measures must be taken to prevent the person from falling.

In dentistry, this is limited but may include cleaning windows or erecting posters on ceilings in the clinical area.
□ Where loft areas are used as store rooms, a fixed ladder, of sound construction and securely fixed, should be provided and maintained.
□ Any changes in levels which are not obvious and could result in people falling should be clearly marked.
□ Objects that are stacked for storage should be positioned in a way that prevents them from falling.

■ **Windows, doors, gates and walls**
□ Transparent fixtures (windows, doors, walls) should be constructed of a safety material or be protected against breakage and marked appropriately.
□ Safety materials (safety glass, plastic sheet) are recommended where fixtures are at shoulder height or below, and at waist height or below.
□ The following dimensions apply to transparent fixtures (*Source: Workplace (Health, Safety and Welfare) ACOP*):
  8 mm thickness – maximum size 1.10 m × 1.10 m
  10 mm thickness – maximum size 2.25 m × 2.25 m
  12 mm thickness – maximum size 3.00 m × 4.50 m
  15 mm thickness – any size
□ All windows should be designed or constructed so that they are capable of being cleaned safely.
□ Doors must be suitably constructed to prevent any type of risk. Examples could be sliding doors from coming off their tracks, rolling doors from falling downwards, powered doors trapping individuals. Powered doors should be capable of being manually operated in case of power failure. Swing doors must provide a clear view of both sides when closed.

■ **Windows, skylights and ventilators**
□ Windows must be capable of being opened and closed without risk to the health and safety of the person carrying out the operation. Windows should not open into an area

where they are likely to present a risk to other persons.

- **Sanitary conveniences (water closets and urinals)**
  - □ Suitable and sufficient facilities should be provided in readily accessible places.
  - □ Areas should be adequately ventilated and lit, maintained in a clean and hygienic condition.
  - □ Separate facilities for men and women may be required if the convenience is not in a separate room and cannot be locked from the inside –for example, if the urinal cannot be sited in a separate area from the toilet used by both sexes.
- **Washing facilities**
  - □ Should be in the immediate vicinity of sanitary conveniences.
  - □ Should be suitable for the workplace and work being undertaken.
  - □ Should have a supply of hot/warm and cold running water, soap/hand cleanser and hygienic suitable drying materials.
  - □ Rooms should be adequately ventilated and lit and maintained in a clean and hygienic condition.
  - □ Showers can be provided if deemed necessary and appropriate.
- **Drinking water**
  - □ Supplies must be fit for human consumption, adequate, situated in accessible places and marked with an appropriate sign confirming that it is safe to drink.
  - □ Suitable cups etc. should also be provided.
  - □ Mains tap water is suitable for human consumption in most workplaces in Great Britain; however, you may have to check with the local water authority.
- **Accommodation and facilities for changing clothing**
  - □ Suitable and sufficient facilities must be provided for people to securely store their personal clothing.
  - □ Work clothing must be stored in a suitable location to prevent the risk of contamination.
  - □ It is recommended in dentistry that personal clothing worn outside of the practice is

removed prior to starting work. Then when leaving work, clinical clothing is removed before leaving the practice. Changing facilities must be accessible, of sufficient space for the number of people using them at any one time and separate facilities should be provided for men and women.

- **Facilities for rest and eating meals**
  - □ Rest areas must have sufficient number of chairs and tables for the number of people using them at any one time.
  - □ Rest areas should be provided where there is no risk of contamination from the work being undertaken, for example, not in the clinical area.
  - □ Rest areas should be provided for nursing and expectant mothers including the facility to lie down, if necessary.
  - □ Eating areas should include facilities for preparing hot and cold food and drinks, for example, a kettle.
  - □ Areas should be maintained in a clean and hygienic condition.
- **Disabled persons**
  - □ The needs of disabled people must be assessed and suitable provisions made to ensure their health, safety and welfare.
  - □ Attention should be given to doors, corridors, stairs, sanitary conveniences, washbasins and workstations.
- **Smoking/tobacco smoke**
  - □ On Sunday, 1 July 2007, England followed the rest of Great Britain and became 'Smokefree'; it is now against the law to smoke in most workplaces throughout England, Ireland, Scotland and Wales.
- **Working at heights**

The relevance of the regulations is limited in dentistry. However, you may identify certain activities which, as previously mentioned, fall under the requirements of the Work at Height Regulations.

Duties placed on employers include the following:

- □ All work is properly planned and organised by competent people.
- □ The risks from working at height are assessed and avoided.

□ Appropriate work equipment is selected, used, maintained and inspected.
□ The risks from fragile surfaces and falling objects are suitably controlled.
□ The need for emergency services in the event of an accident are considered.

Working from home

In certain circumstances, employees may be required to work from home; in these situations, they will be considered to be 'at work'. The employer has a responsibility to protect the employee, just as they would if they were at work in the premises, so far as is reasonably practicable. A suitable and sufficient risk assessment should be undertaken to identify the significant hazards and what must be done to reduce the risk of injury and ill health. The generic risks associated with people who work from home and therefore need to be considered are as follows:

■ Lone working
■ Isolation
■ Safe use of equipment
■ Others who may be in the home, in particular, vulnerable people such as children
■ Rest breaks and working hours
■ Supervision to monitor safety issues
■ Accident reporting and first aid facilities

The analysis of risks will help you determine if it is safe for the employee to work from home or not.

Summary

The health, safety and welfare of all persons should be considered at the design stage of workplaces and revised when adjustments or alterations are being made. Everyone has a responsibility for keeping the working environment in a safe condition. Regular workplace/premises inspections will help to identify the need for rectifications and maintenance to ensure, so far as is reasonable, a safe place.

Action – check the following

■ Do you carry out regular workplace/premises inspections?
■ Do you have a proactive buildings maintenance programme in place?
■ Have you assessed the need for appropriate safety signs and are these communicated effectively?

Frequently asked questions

Q. How many sanitary facilities do we have to provide?
A. The Approved Code of Practice (ACOP) states that the following should be provided based on the maximum number of people likely to be in the workplace at any one time:
□ 1 to 5 people – one WC and one washbasin
□ 6 to 25 people – two WCs and two washbasins
□ 26 to 50 people – three WCs and three washbasins
Where facilities are used only by men the above may differ.
Q. Do we have to provide toilets for visitors/patients?
A. There is no legal requirement for this provision. However, because of the nature of the service provided the health and well-being of clients is extremely important. Therefore it may be advisable to provide the facility. In addition, it may also be a requirement of your contract with the Primary Care Trust (PCT) and also Care Quality Commission in respect of clinical governance.
Q. If someone breaks into our building with the intention of burglary and they are injured can we be held liable?
A. Under the Occupiers Liability Act you are required to take reasonable care for the safety of the public. In this situation, a burglar may be classed as a member of that public. If the occupier is aware that a dangerous condition exists and that a person may be at risk, and nothing has been done about it, then the

burglar, who would be classed as a trespasser, could sue under civil law.

Q. Is there a maximum workplace temperature limit?

A. Not specifically stated; however, reasonable working temperatures should be achieved and maintained. This may require the use of suitable ventilation systems, for example, open doors or windows or air conditioning units.

Q. Do the Work at Height Regulations apply to activities undertaken at less than 1.5 m above ground level?

A. The Regulations have no minimum height requirement as the aim is to prevent injury from falls. Therefore, a risk assessment is required to identify if an activity presents a **significant** risk. In reality, it is unlikely that any activity performed in dentistry will present this level of risk. However, you may want to assess the risk to justify why it is deemed to be a trivial risk.

Links to other chapters

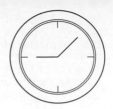

24 Working hours

Scope of this chapter

- Introduction
- Legislation
- Definitions
- Legal limits
- Managing working hours
- Vulnerable groups

Figures

Figure 24.1 – Working Time Regulations 'opt out' record.

Introduction

Excessive and unreasonable working hours can have an adverse effect on an employee's mental and physical health. If employees are suffering from fatigue as a result of their work pattern they are more likely, through the inability to concentrate, to make mistakes which could lead to an accident. In addition, long-term excessive working hours could put undue pressure on individuals, which may lead to work-related stress.

Employers should control working hours so as not to put the health of employees at risk and therefore to prevent accidents. Employers must also ensure that employees are able to make professional judgements and that this process is not impaired by any work place factors under their control.

Legislation

- The Working Time Regulations 1998 (WTR) (as amended):

  Employers have a general duty to ensure that the workforce works appropriate hours with adequate rest and keep records to show that the regulations are being complied with.

- Health and Safety at Work etc. Act 1974:

  Employers must provide and maintain safe systems of work, which are, so far as is reasonably practicable, without risks to health. This covers excessive working hours.

- Disability Discrimination Act 1995 (as amended 2005):

  Employers are required to alter hours of work for disabled persons, where this is deemed to

Managing Health and Safety in the Dental Practice: A Practical Guide, by Jane Bonehill   © 2010 by Blackwell Publishing Ltd.

be necessary and reasonable, to ensure equal employment opportunities.

- Management of Health and Safety at Work Regulations 1999:

  Employers [are] to make suitable and sufficient assessments of risks to health and safety of young persons, new and expectant mothers and any other employee who may be classed as a vulnerable person if subjected to long working hours.

Definitions

Certain phrases are used throughout the Working Time Regulations 1998 (WTR) as defined below:

- Working time – working for an employer, carrying out his activities and duties, including periods of training. Travel to work is not classed as working time, however, and employers will need to agree to what constitutes working time for workers who travel as part of their job.
- Worker – a person undertaking any duties or activities under a contract of employment whether this is in writing or verbal. This might be a person who is paid a salary or where someone works under a different contract of employment, where, for example, the employer provides the worker with equipment and health and safety controls to do the job and pays the worker's tax and national insurance contributions.
- Young person/worker – in England and Wales, a worker who is over the compulsory minimum school leaving age and under the age of 18 years, and in Scotland over the school leaving age.

Legal limits

Enforcement

Enforcement of the WTR is split between two authorities as follows:

- Health and Safety Executive (and others for specific industries) will enforce legal working limits.
- Employment Tribunals will enforce the entitlements for rest periods and annual leave.

Legal limits

Legal limits provide the rights for people at work. They also cover those who work for an agency who may have a different type of contract. Legal limits differ for adults and young persons and are specified as follows:

- **Weekly working time:**
  - Adults – maximum of 48 hours in each 7-day period averaged over a 17-week period. This limit will cover most dental professionals. However, this can be extended to a 26-week period in certain circumstances, most of which are likely to be irrelevant in dentistry.
  - Maximum working hours can be extended if an 'opt out' agreement is drawn up between employer and employee.
  - Young persons – must not work more than 8 hours per day and a maximum of 40 hours per week.
- **Rest periods:**
  Weekly:
  - Adults – are entitled to an uninterrupted rest break of 24 hours (1 day) in each 7-day period.
  - Young persons – are entitled to an uninterrupted rest break of 48 hours (2 days) in each 7-day period.
  Daily:
  - Adults – 11 consecutive hours rest in any 24-hour period (within each working day).
  - Young persons – 12 consecutive hours rest in any 24-hour period (within each working day).
  In work:
  - Adults – if they work for longer than 6 hours they are entitled to a minimum of 20 minutes uninterrupted break away from their work area. This should be organised, so that it is taken during the 6 hours and not at the beginning or end.

- Young persons – if they work for longer than 4.5 hours are entitled to a minimum of 30 minutes uninterrupted break away from their work area. This should be taken in one session of 30 minutes.
- **Annual leave:**
  - From 1 October 2007, the WTR was amended to extend the annual leave entitlement to 24 days paid annual leave per year after 13 weeks employment. Prior to the amendment the entitlement was 4 weeks/20 days. In both cases, the employer could incorporate the eight bank holidays into the entitlement.
  - From 1 April 2009, the WTR was further amended to extend the annual leave entitlement to 28 days paid annual leave per year including bank holidays.
  - Paid leave is calculated on the basis of the number of days per week a person works and is calculated on a pro rata basis for part-time staff.

Managing working hours

- Employers should keep records of working hours for each employee to ensure compliance with the regulations. Records could be simple time sheets or existing formats used by the organisation such as pay slips.
- Employers must ensure that workers do not exceed the legal working limits by calculating and analysing working hours and patterns.
- If overtime is required employers must establish if this means that overall hours will exceed the legal limit and then assess the risk to the employee and if necessary make a justifiable case for detracting from the regulations. If this is likely to be a recurring occurrence then...
- The employer may need to formalise the fact that some employees will regularly exceed the legal limit and draw up an 'opt out' agreement. This must be employee-led and ultimately be his/her decision. The employee must sign to say that he/she agrees to exceeding the working limits (Figure 24.1).
- Employers must arrange appointment systems and work schedules to ensure that in work rest periods can be taken.

- Employers should check that staff take their daily and weekly breaks and if there is reason to believe that additional work/employment is being undertaken, discuss the options – for example, reducing their hours or obtaining an 'opt out' agreement.
- Employers should manage annual leave by determining employees' entitlement, organising leave schedules and monitoring staff to ensure that they are taking the required amount of days.
- Employers should identify those people who may be more at risk, make a suitable and sufficient assessment and implement the necessary controls.

Vulnerable groups

Certain groups of workers may be more vulnerable and therefore more at risk from excessive working hours because of their individual circumstances. Those listed below are relevant to dental environments.

- Working for more than one employer – it is likely that the weekly limit will be exceeded and therefore could adversely affect the individual's health, safety and well-being.
- New and expectant mothers – may be more at risk if they work longer hours as they are likely to have disturbed sleep patterns and conditions associated with pregnancy.
- Home workers – in certain circumstances, employees, in particular, practice managers, may be required to work from home. In these situations, they will be considered to be 'at work'; it is not always possible to monitor the hours of work and rest periods.
- On-call workers – this mainly applies to on-call staff in a hospital setting. However, it could also apply to dental staff who provide the emergency on-call service. The working time does not start until they are called upon by their employer.
- Disabled workers – may not be able to cope with excessive hours because of their individual condition.

- Young persons – because of their inexperience or work patterns and workplace demands. The limits described in this chapter are an absolute must and the young person cannot decide to extend these limits (exceptions are allowed).

Legal working limits should not be exceeded for any worker. The above list is intended to highlight additional reasons for ensuring compliance for those who may be more at risk.

Summary

Employers should eliminate the need for people to work long hours and look at ways to change working patterns. Working smarter and having flexible working arrangements will motivate the workforce and help in achieving the work–life balance.

Action – check the following

- Have you calculated how many hours a week each individual works?
- Do you have a means of recording working hours for all employees?
- Do you ensure that staff take the required in work rest periods?

Frequently asked questions

Q. Can an employee exceed the legal working hours?

Figure 24.1   Working Time Regulations 'opt out' record.

By completing the first four columns of this form you are agreeing to exceed the legal weekly working limits of 48 hours. If at any time you want to terminate the agreement you must give the required notice period and complete the fifth column.

Name of employee	Job title	Signature	Date of agreement	Date of terminating agreement and signature

A. In certain circumstances, an employee may decide to work more than 48 hours per week for his/her employer. A written agreement must be in place which applies to a specified period or indefinitely and can be terminated by the employee, provided notice is given. Notice can be given with a minimum of 7 days and up to a period of 3 months. This is sometimes referred to as an *opt out agreement* and can only apply to weekly working limit. Young persons cannot opt out and if the employee has more than one employer the 'opt out' must be agreed to by both/all. The employer must keep a record of employees who have an 'opt out' agreement.

Q. If an employee wants to receive additional pay in lieu of some of his/her annual leave is this permissible?

A. No, employees must take 4 weeks' paid annual leave.

Q. The practice opens for 12 hours per day, 6 days a week. When we experience staff shortages we ask staff to work overtime. Is this allowed?

A. Flexibility with working hours is allowed in certain circumstances, in particular, where there are unexpected and unforeseen occurrences. However, if this is a routine occurrence then you may want to determine the need for an 'opt out' agreement or alternative measures, for example, contracting with an agency to provide temporary/locum cover.

Links to other chapters

Chapter 11 – Lone working
Chapter 15 – Occupational health and well-being
Chapter 20 – Stress management

Sources of advice and information

Access Disability Ltd – www.accessdisability.co.uk

Advisory, Conciliation and Arbitration Service (ACAS) – www.acas.org.uk

British Association of Dental Nurses (BADN) – www.badn.org.uk

British Dental Association (BDA) – www.bda.org

Care Quality Commission – www.cqc.org.uk

Criminal Records Bureau – www.crb.homeoffice.gov.uk

Department For Environment, Food and Rural Affairs (DEFRA) – www.defra.gov.uk

DenMed Training and Consultancy – www.denmed-uk.com

Department of Health (DOH) – www.doh.gov.uk

Department of Trade and Industry (DTI) – www.dti.gov

Disability Rights Commission (DRC) – www.ODI.gov.uk

Health Protection Agency (HPA) – www.hpa.org.uk

Health and Safety Executive (HSE) – www.hse.gov.uk

Incident Contact Centre, Caerphilly Business Centre, Caerphilly Business Park, Caerphilly, CF83 3GG Email to mailto:riddor@connaught.plc.uk or fax to 0845 300 9924 (for Reporting an injury or dangerous occurrence)

Independent Safeguarding Authority – www.isa.gov.org.uk

Institution of Occupational Safety and Health (IOSH) – www.iosh.co.uk

Medicines and Healthcare products Regulatory Agency (MHRA) – www.mhra.gov.uk

National Health Service (NHS) – www.nhs.uk

National Statistics Office – www.statistics.gov.uk

Index